BLONDIE WITHOUT BORDERS

CHRISTINE SEIBOLD

Table of Contents

DEDICATION:

To all of those women who have ever thought you weren't enough, you were, you are, and you always will be.

Merriam Webster's Definitions:

Boundary (n)

bound·ary | \ ˈbau̇n-d(ə-)rē \

Definition of *boundary:*

something that indicates or fixes a limit or extent

Border (n)

bor·der | \ ˈbȯr-dər \

Definition of *border*

an outer part or edge; boundary

MY WHY

I am writing this book for two main reasons. First, my grandfather was a writer, who shared his stories and inspired my father to be a writer, who has now inspired me to write.

When my grandfather died, my family found numerous books and stories that he had written that were never published. My dad also used to write poems and journals and has published some articles and a couple of chapters in a book. I am writing this book so that I can become the first member of my family that has published a complete book.

My second "why" for writing this book is to help get my message across about the importance of boundaries and what happens in life when there are none.

I am writing it to share all the difficult circumstances that I have fought through and overcome in my life. I want to show women that no matter what you go through, you can always move forward. You can always get through to the other side. There is always a little bit of hope.

I want women to know that they are enough just the way they are. It is also ok to set boundaries in relationships, with work, with self-care, with money, with food, with alcohol, and whatever else may cross your path. It is ok to say no, and it is ok to not feel guilty about saying no.

INTRODUCTION

Hi, how are you? I'm Christine, but my family and close friends call me Chris and Christy. I am going to let you in on a little secret. Ready for it...! I am not a natural blonde! I have been a blonde for the last 20 years of my life, but I am a natural brunette.

Thank you for reading my memoir. I have worked hard to share my stories, examples and lessons learned from my life that will hopefully resonate with you. Perhaps they will give you some areas to reflect on with regards to setting boundaries and why they are so important.

All the stories in the book are true life stories. I have changed the names and some of the roles of the characters to protect everyone's identity in the story, except my own. So let's get started!

My whole life, I have been on a journey to find love. I can remember the first crush that I had on my classmate, Matty Jones, all the way back in preschool. I have always longed to feel that special love from another man. That is not to say that my father and mother don't love me; they love me very much and I have learned what true, unconditional love is from them. But it is a different kind of love that I have always yearned for. I have longed for a deeper connection with someone that I can trust completely and share all my secrets with. That fairytale kind of love that you see in the movies.

Matty Jones and I finished pre-school and ended up in the same grammar school. When we started Kindergarten, I still had a crush on Matty. I dreamed of growing older with him and having a happy ever after wedding with the story of the two of us who met in pre-school and loved each other our whole lives. But at the same time, I found that I also had a crush on an 8th grader named Charlie when I was in Kindergarten. That's right, I was 5 and he was 13! Something in me was not right, but I thought that Charlie was SO HOT! I remember getting in trouble with my parents after a sleepover with my Kindergarten bestie because my parents found homemade drawings made by yours truly, that were asking Charlie to have sex with me. As if I knew what that meant at 5 years old!

I went to a Catholic grammar school and it was always the same story. Whoever I had a crush on never seemed to like me back. It was always a struggle to find love. Charlie graduated from the eighth grade and went on to high school. Eventually after the third grade, Matty left my grammar school and transferred to the local public school. That pretty much ended any kind of relationship that we had. We stayed in touch over the years, and I was heartbroken when I discovered that Matty was hit by a car crossing the street when we were 14 years old. I will never forget the night my parents told me. I had a really hard time getting over that tragedy and the fact that my "first love" was truly gone and I would never talk to him again. Matty was dead which meant I would never have that fairy tale wedding with him.

My first peck on the lips happened when I was 12 at a birthday party with my classmate Scott Powers. To this day, I still have a scar on my knee from when I ran into the rock that we went behind to have the kiss. I mean they say love hurts, right? I think we were together for about two weeks when he dumped me for another girl in our class. Oh, the heartache!

When I was 13, I dated my friend Christian, who lived a few streets over from me. Christian had just moved to Massachusetts from out of state and was new in my school. As one of the nerds in my class, I was asked to go to his house a few days a week to help him catch up with the lessons as a new student and "help" him with homework. But all we would really do is go to his room and make out! I remember the day when my parents found the note I had written to my classmate Samantha telling her that Christian and I had French kissed. Needless to say, that did not go over well with my parents and they forbid me to go to Christian's house anymore to study.

I'll never forget how nervous I was in eighth grade when I told my mother the first time that I was "going out" with Michael Stan. It was early one morning as she was dropping me off at school. My whole body was tense and full of fear for the 15-minute car ride from home to school. As she pulled into the parking lot, my body froze because I didn't know what she would say or what her reaction would be. I knew she thought I was too young to be going to dances, so I didn't expect a positive reaction from her when I told her about my new boyfriend.

My mother didn't even know what "going out" meant. Neither did I, but I knew that it gave me this warm tingly feeling when I received attention and love from Michael. Michael was immature and always farting and telling silly jokes. I mean, that is what eighth graders do, isn't it? I didn't really love him, but it felt good to "have a boyfriend" like some of the other girls in my class. We stayed together for about a year, but we broke up when we decided to attend different high schools. We kept in contact after we went to high school since Michael lived about 7 minutes down the road from me. Sadly, in our sophomore year of high school, Michael died in a drunk driving accident when he ran into a telephone pole. He died immediately from the impact. The whole thing was so sad, and again, I had lost another love of mine.

The summer before high school, I had developed a very special relationship with my cousin, Al, on a family vacation trip. He was a couple of years younger than me and lived out in the state of Nevada. From the first moment we met, we developed a tight bond. We instantly became glued to each other. We shared a best-friend type of love and really understood each other. We used to write letters back and forth and send them in the mail. We would talk on the phone for hours and share our deepest darkest secrets.

And then one evening I was woken up by the answering machine, which we kept in our guest bedroom. I have always been a light sleeper, and one night, I kept hearing a beeping noise, so I got up to see what it was. I went into the guest room and realized we had a voicemail. When I pressed the play button, I almost fainted. My uncle, Al's father and my dad's brother, had left a message on the answering machine saying that Al had died in a car accident around the corner from their house. I did not know what to do. I held onto the desk as I almost fell over. It couldn't be true; I must have heard him wrong. I played the message again, but I had heard correctly the first time. There, on the answering machine, was my uncle's sad voice telling us that Al had had an accident and didn't make it. I burst into tears and fell to the ground. I couldn't believe it, and I ran downstairs to my parent's bedroom to tell them.

Al's death was the third loss of a man who I truly cared about deeply, before I turned 23. Al was closer to me than anyone else in the world, and he was gone. One thing that I did learn very early from Matty, Michael, and Al's losses was that life is precious and can end at any time. From their losses, I gained the mentality to live life to the fullest, because you never know when it will be over. Losing Matty, Michael, and Al at a young age gave me even more of a desire to find true love and to live each day as if it is my last.

My first "real love" as a teenager was with Earl. You will learn more about him later, but he was my friend's older brother and was two years older than me. We met shortly before I turned 16, and I thought for sure he was the one. But he wasn't. And that pattern went on for years. I thought he was the one, but he wasn't. *Maybe love wasn't really for me,* I often thought.

As I grew into my 20s, I became one of those serial daters. I longed to be and feel genuinely loved, so I was always in a committed relationship or seeing somebody, even if he wasn't the best person for me. Why couldn't I just be alone? Why did I always have to have a boyfriend? I never even learned who I was as a person because I was always learning to conform to be like whoever it was that I was dating. If he liked rock music, then I liked rock. If he liked country, then I was a country fan and in the front row at the country fest concert in the summer at Gillette Stadium.

My serial dating turned into countless men. Some of them you will learn about in this book. I am grateful for all the experiences that I have gone through with all my relationships, good and bad, because they have brought me to where I am today.

Today, I am happily married to Anderson, a healthy, beautiful, kind man with whom I have an amazing relationship. He supports me and loves me no matter what. With him, I experience true, unconditional love, both with him and from him, and I am so grateful for that. It is amazing to have someone love me for all of my traits, the good and the bad, and who accepts all of me, just as I am. I guess you can say, I finally have found my fairytale man.

But the journey to finding love has not been easy. Sometimes I look back and think to myself, *How are you still alive?*

Some of the stories that you will read ahead are unbelievable, but they are all true and they all happened to me. I honestly believe we are put on this earth for a reason, whether it is to teach and influence others with our message or to help others in another way. I hope my stories help you, make you laugh, and teach you an invaluable lesson. Know that it is never too late to improve or change whatever you may want in your life. You can be anyone you want to be, and do anything you want to do. It is never too late to start. Most importantly, it is ok to say "no" and set boundaries if something or someone is not good for you.

With all that being said, getting to a place where I can set healthy boundaries and believe that I can do anything has only come after years of therapy and hard work on myself. Only then could I get to a place where I completely love all of who I am. And so I encourage you to do the same. Love yourself, and you can do anything you want.

CHRONOLOGY OF CHRISTINE

1982: November 30, 4:28 PM Christine Rose Seibold was born into this world in Worcester, Massachusetts.

1986: Christine was told by her pre-school teacher, Mrs. G., that she needed to learn how to use her inside voice. (I like to think that I was already in training to be a strong woman who just wanted to be heard.)

1994: I had my first kiss in 6th grade with Scott Powers at a birthday party. (I still have the scar on my knee from when I fell and hit a rock to prove it.)

1996: I lost my first crush, Matty Jones, to a car accident as he was crossing the street.

1998: I lost my 8th grade boyfriend, Michael Stan, to a car crash not too far from home. I also met Patty and Mik, my two best friends to this day.

2001: I graduated from St. Peter Marian High School in Worcester, Massachusetts, and I went to The College of Saint Rose in Albany, New York.

2003-2004: I left the United States for the first time (besides visiting Canada) to travel abroad to Seville, Spain. I loved it so much in 2003 that I found a way to study abroad there again in 2004.

2005: I graduated from the College of Saint Rose with a double degree in Spanish and Public Communications. I also lost my cousin Al late that fall in a car crash and was completely devastated.

2005: I got married to my first husband, Walter.

2008: Walter and I got divorced.

2009: I got sober for the first time and did a lot of inside work on myself.

2011: I moved back to Seville, Spain to teach English for two years.

2012: I got sober for the second time after a 5-day relapse and have been sober since then (yay!)

2013: I got married to my second husband Ahmed after leaving Spain and moving back to Boston.

2016: I divorced Ahmed after his verbal and emotional abuse turned physical. I did not date for a year and did a lot of therapy and soul searching.

2017: I met Anderson, my third and FINAL husband. He is amazing, supportive, and loves me unconditionally for exactly who I am.

2018: I graduated with my Master's degree from Harvard University in International Relations. I also moved with Anderson from Boston to Miami, Florida in the fall. I started my own business, Freelance N' Freedom.

2020: I founded Femprendedoras, a women's membership community of learning and mutual support for entrepreneurial women in Seville, Spain. I love these women. They were my heart and strength during Covid.

2021: I married Anderson, the love of my life, on June 25th at my best friend Mik's house in Newburyport, MA. It was a beautiful day of celebration full of love and happiness.

CAPÍTULO UNO: THE RAIN IN SPAIN STAYS MAINLY ON THE PLAIN

The day is finally here! There is nothing that I enjoy more in this world than to travel. When I say travel, I don't mean actually going through the airport and getting on an airplane. I HATE planes and can never fall asleep or get comfortable on them. What I am referring to is the excitement and adventure that comes with seeing a new place for the first time and not knowing what to expect. It is that feeling when you get to the top of a mountain or volcano and think, *Whoa! Did I just climb up here?* I love seeing beautiful cities, trying new food, and hearing and seeing new languages and places (like Iceland or New Zealand) that make you feel like you are on another planet.

I have traveled to 60 countries, and right now, I am overjoyed with excitement because I have waited so long to take my husband, Anderson, to my favorite place in the world: Seville, Spain. Spain was the first country I visited outside of the United States (besides Canada). Ever since I was a little girl, I always wanted to speak Spanish and visit Spain. I thought it was so cool to be able to speak another language, and to be able to connect with people from different cultures. Of course, I also thought of the benefits of having a conversation that other people didn't understand!

My dream finally came true when I studied in Sevilla for a semester in college in 2003. I loved it so much that I went back a year later to do a second semester in the spring of 2004. Later, I returned in 2011-2013 to teach English in the Spanish grammar school system. Of the 60 countries I have traveled to, and the thousands of cities I have visited, Seville is by far my favorite place in the world. There is even a song called *"Sevilla tiene un color especial,"* which means "Seville has a special color about it," and that is nothing but true.

Seville is the third largest city in Spain, and the capital of Andalusia, the region that makes up the south of Spain. It is filled with beautiful parks, the third largest cathedral in the world, the Guadalquivir River, a castle, Moorish architecture, horse carts and buggies, and small cobblestone streets that wind throughout the city.

The center is filled with quaint little shops and restaurants with patios outside. People are constantly walking in the center with their families, dressed in their Sunday best, enjoying the pleasant weather. Andalusia is known for having 300 plus days of sunshine and extremely warm summers. In August, the cities shut down, and everyone goes to the beach. And let's not forget the most beautiful part of Seville: the *Plaza de España*. That is where they filmed part of the *Star Wars* movie. It is just the most magnificent magical breathtaking place that I have ever been, and I never get tired of visiting it.

I have wanted more than anything to take the man that I love to this amazing city for years, but the government has not made that possible until now. Even when I met Anderson, I tried to set a boundary with him when I told him that I was moving back to Spain and warned him that we'd better not get into a serious relationship.

I had applied to go back and teach English in Seville again before I met Anderson, and I did not want to let a man get in the way. As you can see, that worked really well! We ended up falling for each other quickly, and I gave away my spot in the English teaching program to stay in Boston with Anderson until he could legally travel.

Seeing that Anderson is from Brazil, and the administration under President Trump had been nothing but unfavorable towards immigrants, the process of renewing his papers to be legal in the United States was an exceedingly long, painful, expensive, and complicated process. However, now that the process is over, it is time to go together to this magical city, where the warmth from the sunshine is infectious, the tapas are tasty and cheap, and the smell of the orange trees and Azahar (a beautiful Spanish flower that grows on trees) fills your nostrils as you walk down the street.

Ever since date three, Anderson told me he was on board with moving to Spain with me to give our relationship a shot. Our connection was instantaneous, and it has never faltered since. Our chemistry was clear from the start. When I told him on our second date that I was planning on moving back to Spain, he came back on date three and showed me how much personal trainers could make in Spain. This was him indicating that he was with me on this and that he would go wherever I went, as long as we could be together.

A part of me now wonders what it will be like to go back. The last time I was in Seville, I was living with my horrible ex, Ahmed, who was my fiancé at the time. Ahmed was from Casablanca, Morocco and had a vastly different view of the world than I did. I met Ahmed in 2012 when I was teaching English in Seville. We moved home to the United States against my will in the summer of 2013, because there were no jobs for him in Spain and I could not support the both of us. I wanted to stay in Spain teaching, but the reality of him as an immigrant finding work in Seville during the economic crisis was slim to none. He had already been unemployed there for two years as a student, and with the teacher's salary I was making, I could not support the both of us long-term. So we decided it would be best to apply for the fiancé visa and move back to the states to get married. He proposed to me next to the Eiffel Tower on my 30th birthday, and I said yes.

During the time that we dated, we would argue and fight quite often, and I should have known early on that our relationship would not work. We would fight about cultural differences, as he grew up Muslim and I grew up Catholic. Spiritually, what was important to me was that we both believed in God. He told me that that was what was important to him too, but it turned out he wasn't telling me the truth.

Even though we had spoken about it many times, soon after our wedding, he told me that he wanted me to convert to be Muslim. For him, everything that he did was based on Islam, and he thought that I should also base my actions on his religion too. As you can imagine, this caused a lot of tension within our marriage and was hard because he wanted me to change who I was for him.

Unfortunately, the situation did not end well, and it took the four T's—therapy, tears, travel, and time—to get over the difficult marriage. I was left scarred after my relationship with him, and I began questioning who I was as a woman and who had I become (more on that later). Would it be difficult to go back and visit Sevilla again? Would I be constantly reliving the memories that Ahmed and I had from there?

I have worked hard over the years at forgiving myself for the poor decisions that I made when it came to Ahmed. I should have listened to those around me who had seen us together and said we were not a match… but I didn't. I should have listened to my sisters, who saw us fighting all the time when they came to visit us; they had told me that he was closed off and unfriendly to them… but I didn't. I should have listened to my two best friends, Mik and Patty, who said he was negative and nasty… but I ignored them too. Most importantly, I should have listened to myself. I did not listen to that little voice inside of me saying, *Give it more time. Just wait. Don't leave the place you love for this man…* but I didn't.

And I'm okay with that today. All the difficult experiences that followed my exit from Sevilla led me to where I am today. I am happier than I have ever been in my whole 38 years on earth. Sure, I wouldn't have minded saving myself from heartache, stress, depression, abuse, and pain. But then again, those situations made me a strong, confident woman, who became clear on who she is for once in her life and what she wants. And I wouldn't have met Anderson, the love of my life, if I had stayed in Spain at that time. Everything happens for a reason. At least, that is what I believe.

So, as we board the plane and get ready to take off, I take Anderson's hand and look him in the eyes. I am so excited for our first international trip together and eager to see what he thinks about my favorite city in the world. *Will he love it as much as I do? What if he doesn't want to move here in the future?* So many questions are flooding my head as the plane takes off down the runway in Miami.

CAPÍTULO DOS: I ATE IT! I HATE IT!

We arrived in Spain with no problems. The flight to Madrid was smooth, and the transition to Seville was quick and easy. I didn't sleep a wink on the plane, but that was nothing new. Between the minimal legroom and the excitement inside of me, I stayed up all night watching movies.

After we collected our bags at the airport, we snapped a selfie in front of the *"Bienvenida a Sevilla"* sign. I was happy to have learned that Seville has Uber now, which they did not have when I lived there before. Uber made it much easier to get out of the airport and into the city without getting ripped off by the taxi drivers.

Since our flight was overnight, we pulled into the hotel at around 9:30 a.m. Breakfast at the hotel was included in our room rate. *Yesssssssss,* I thought to myself. I always loved it when the buffet at the hotel was all-you-can-eat.

After unpacking some of our things, we went downstairs to the cafe for breakfast. The Spanish spread was unbelievable! They had the typical Spanish tostadas with local olive oil, ham, and tomato paste. There was also a German breakfast layout with vegetables, cheese, and sausage, and then you had an American type of breakfast with pancakes, bacon, and eggs. At the end by the coffee machine, there were also a bunch of homemade Spanish croissants and pastries to choose from.

I loaded up my plate and made sure to grab some of the pastries at the end of the line. *Oh, how I have missed the tostadas and the cafes con leche! This is going to be AMAZING*, I thought.

As I brought the Spanish muffin to my mouth, it brought me back to a time when I was really struggling with food addiction.

As I reached into the package of chocolate chip cookies, I grabbed my fifth one and brought it to my mouth. *My fifth cookie!* I thought to myself. *How could this be? I just opened them!*

The realization that yet, once again, I had overindulged in a "bad" food that I should not be eating right now settled into my brain. Immediately, shame and negative thoughts flooded my head: *You're so fat and ugly! There you go again, you loser! How could you be so stupid? You are going to gain 10 more pounds from those cookies you just ate!*

I was stuck in my own head and couldn't escape my negative thoughts and terrible feelings (once again) as I looked down and stared at my bloated stomach that stuck out of my t-shirt. Unfortunately, this pattern of binge-eating sweets had become almost a daily habit.

I grew up the oldest of three in an Irish Catholic family in a small town, west of Boston, Massachusetts. My parents were hardworking providers that came from very little. They did everything they could to make sure that my younger twin sisters and I had a good life. Along with that came many hours of dedication and hard work. I am grateful to my parents for instilling a great work ethic in me today. However, many hours of hard work also meant that my sisters and I were often at home being taken care of by someone else.

Mabel was a strong, Irish-Catholic woman, who I never saw cry during the 15 years of my life that she took care of my sisters and me. She taught me that I should treat others with love and respect and to be caring and generous. Unfortunately, and contradictory to what she told me; she did not live by those same words.

Mabel was a woman of the church. She was generous in donating money to various charities and poor children in China. But for some reason, she greatly favored my younger sisters over me. She treated me very poorly, yelled at me, locked me in dark spaces, and scolded me for things that I did not even do. She would slap me around, wash my mouth out with soap, and make me clean the floor with a toothbrush whenever she considered me to be a "bad girl." She would play mind games with me and give me copies of the Golden Rule or the Girl Scout Law and would order me to memorize them so I could become a "better person" when I was 8 years old.

Every time that I was being yelled at, or I felt uncomfortable, or was being told that I was a horrible sister, I turned to food. Each time that I was upset with something Mabel did, I asked her for food. Mabel would laugh in my face and say, "Where does all this food go? You must have a hollow leg!" Needless to say, she would give me endless pieces of toast and other snacks, probably to just shut me up.

I learned as a young child that food was my best friend. It gave me comfort and made me feel better in my moments of hurt and sadness. I cherished it as if it were my soulmate, something that I longed for and needed to get through the day. Those days turned into weeks, and those weeks turned into years. And that was the beginning with my boundaryless relationship with food.

My parents firmly believed in getting a Catholic education. My sisters and I went to a private Catholic school from kindergarten to 8th grade and then high school and college as well. I was always tall for my age and an awkwardly shaped teenager. I sprouted to my 5-foot 9 height by seventh grade, which made me tower over all the other girls and even most of the boys in my class. Of course, this made me feel huge! I played soccer from the age of 5 until I was 18, and naturally, being tall, I played basketball in junior high and high school.

Something inside me always made me feel out of place. I was always somewhat chubby, although looking back, I was taller than fat, but I didn't realize it at the time. In my mind, I always felt huge, and for whatever reason, I equated my size with my self-worth as a person. In junior high, I was always teased and made fun of by the other girls in my class. I tried so hard to fit in, but they always found some reason to laugh at me. In high school, I was never the "popular" one, and I lacked a lot of confidence from my experience with the girls in junior high. I also ended up attending a high school that had a middle school attached, and 90% of my class already knew each other and had formed close bonds since 7th grade.

Every morning when I got to my high school, I would buy a Snickers bar (or two) from the vending machine in the cafeteria. Snickers would keep me safe and calm my nerves. *Snickers, the breakfast of champions,* I thought as I rolled my eyes at myself. Snickers was my second breakfast, of course, because I had already eaten at home.

I remember one particular day when I arrived at school, I went up to the vending machine to buy my daily Snickers. I returned to where my friends were sitting to listen in on the conversation. As I stood, I leaned over the wastebasket. Before I knew it, my Snickers bar had fallen out of the wrapper and into the wastebasket!

"Oh no!" I said as I looked at my girlfriends. I didn't have any more money that day, and I HAD to eat that candy bar. *How am I going to get through the day without my Snickers,* I thought.

I stared at my friends, and then looked into the trash. When I looked at the trash, I noticed that the bag was new and had been recently changed since it was early in the morning. I bent down and grabbed the candy bar out of the trash.

"Ewwwwwwww!" I heard my friends say as I picked it up. "Tell me you are NOT going to eat that… Are you?!" they asked me.

I stood there and contemplated what to say to them. Of course, I was going to eat it. I HAD to eat it. How would I get through my morning without my Snickers?

I smiled, took a bite, and told them, "The trash bag was just changed. Look!" as I pointed down to the bag. My friends started laughing at me, and looked at me with strange faces, but I didn't care.

By the time I got to college, I was at the point where I couldn't bring myself to step on the scale, but I for sure was well over 250 pounds. I attended a small private college in Albany, New York, called The College of Saint Rose.

Earl, my boyfriend of three years, and the reason that I left Boston to go to school in Albany, had just dumped me for another girl. We ended up splitting shortly after I started college there, even though we had kept a successful long-distance relationship for 2 years when he left for college. I was truly heartbroken and did everything I could to get him back, but it did not work out. With all the emotional turmoil, as I had done in the past, I turned to food.

Food became my go-to "friend" to turn to for comfort ever since that young age and my experiences with Mabel. It was like it was a part of me. When I had something to celebrate, I turned to food. When I went through a bad breakup or my horrible divorce, I turned to food. When I lost my dog, I turned to food. When I was unhappy at my job, food was there again. This unhealthy pattern would always turn into gaining back whatever weight I had lost from whatever diet I was on at the time.

Finally, when I separated from my first husband and was tired of my weight and the way I looked, I gave Weight Watchers a try and I lost 80 pounds. In 2009, after I got sober, I became an avid runner and started running full marathons. This helped me keep the weight off for years, but then it eventually started to creep back up when I stopped running. I couldn't eat the number of calories that I had when I would run every day. I soon found myself back over 200 pounds again.

At around the age of 30 when I was teaching English in Spain, I finally became aware that I had an issue and was bingeing on food. I had been sober from alcohol for a little over three years, and I realized that I had been using food as a substitute for alcohol to fill the void when I had stopped drinking.

Living in Spain, I found myself going to the store and buying large amounts of groceries. I would eat cookies, cakes, chips, and anything that I thought would make me feel better, until I was really stuffed. This soon became a habit, and I would become irritable and cranky if I could not get the food I wanted when I wanted it. I never had the guts to throw it up. I tried once after bingeing on an ice cream sundae, but it did not work and resulted in horrible feelings about myself, so I never did it again.

A girl from Massachusetts who was studying abroad in Spain told me about a recovery program back home that her mom did. The program was called Food Addicts Anonymous. It was like AA, but for food instead of alcohol. She told me the whole point of the program was to eat 3 meals a day only, eliminate flour and sugar, and to weigh and measure everything that went in your mouth. I decided that I was done with bingeing (for now), and before I moved home from Spain, I started to eliminate as much flour and sugar from my diet as possible. To my surprise, I started to lose weight.

When I moved back home to Boston in 2013, I found FA meetings and started attending. It turned out, after a couple of stabs at FA, that it was extremely strict and not for me, so I decided to leave, even though I had lost a good amount of weight fast. There were too many rules and boundaries, and I found myself bingeing even more due to the restrictions. This only resulted in feeling bad for myself and shame after I binged. I did not feel I could live a balanced healthy life in that program, so I left.

Today, I am happy to say that I have a much healthier relationship and boundaries with food. I can't even remember the last time I binged. I have worked with a Fitness Coach, who also touches on the mental aspect of food. The goal was to clear away any beliefs and ideas that I had around food that started back when I was younger that had become ingrained in me and almost automatic. I exercise along with a healthy diet and eat healthy foods that make me feel good about myself. Through this I have lost a great deal of weight. I have also worked hard with a counselor to get rid of the negative thinking and self-talk, which has helped tremendously.

LESSONS LEARNED

No amount of food can fill a void and make a situation better. I had to work from the inside out to deal with my food issues and past trauma in order to find peace with food and myself. Health is not something to be taken for granted. You are enough and do not need any food or any substance to change who you are. Treat yourself and your body with kindness, and love yourself. You are worth it!

CAPÍTULO TRES: THE CALL OF ALCOHOL/ THE FALL OF ALCOHOL

Warning. Difficult information in this chapter.

After breakfast, I took Anderson out into the city. I was so excited that I could feel the adrenaline pumping. We walked through the center and across the river into my old neighborhood. I wanted to show him where I used to live in Los Remedios, one of the neighborhoods in Seville. I actually had lived in that neighborhood for quite some time. The first time was in 2003 when I lived with a host family when I studied abroad. I was assigned to a family that lived in Los Remedios and also lived with a roommate from Bosnia.

The second time I lived there was the first year that I taught English in Seville when I returned in 2011. I had found roommates that had a small room available, and since I knew the neighborhood from my previous time there, I decided to take it. I liked living there because of its proximity to the *Feria de Abril* fairgrounds (a Spanish flamenco festival that happens every year in April) and also to Calle Betis, where all the bars were located.

We walked over the bridge, across the river, and into the Plaza de Cuba. I noticed the metal bars on the bridge were still filled with locks of love from couples who had written their initials and attached them to the metal bars. I may or may not have participated in this silly ritual with a guy or two back in the day. I chuckled to myself as we passed by the locks.

As we walked into the Plaza de Cuba and down Calle Betis, a wave of emotion came about me. Calle Betis was known as the "party street" where the *güiris* (Spanish slang for foreigners) frequently hung out. I certainly had spent many nights there. Some I remember, and others I do not.

The street ran along the river and was the connector between the Los Remedios neighborhood and Triana. This was the neighborhood in Seville where flamenco began. It was a colorful little street with bar after bar. There were bars with rock music, bars with flamenco shows, and bars with hip hop/pop music. It was filled with promoters who were trying to get *güiris* to come inside their bar by handing out free shots and buy-one/get-one-free tickets.

Many of the bars even had names that appealed to foreigners like *The Long Island Bar*, *The Second Room,* and *Fun Club.* Walking by Fun Club caused me to have flashbacks. I suddenly had memories of throwing up outside of Fun Club while I leaned on one of the orange trees and flashbacks of walking home wasted, out of control, and out of my mind.

I will never forget the first time that I took a drink and alcohol touched my lips. I was instantly in love. I was 16 years old at a house party with my friend, Laura, from high school. The homeowner was my boyfriend Earl's best friend at the time. Earl was two years older than me and had already been drinking beers on the weekends for quite some time. The warm fuzzy bitterness was a foreign taste, but it went down so easily. I felt so light and happy after a few sips, and I totally understood why people loved drinking. Laura had an older boyfriend too and had already tried beer and had been drunk a couple of times, so it was nothing new to her. She was happy to tag along to a party that had free beer.

Earl was in a fraternity at his college in Albany, and so, as most fraternities do, they had lots of parties. I would go up and visit Earl every few weeks with my best friend, Patty. We loved the adventure of driving up there, being social, and getting tipsy or drunk every time we went. Even though we were not 21 yet, it was quite easy to get alcohol from the fraternity members. Additionally, they often paid for us if we went out. We loved the adventure and the mystery of where the night and the alcohol would take us (more to come on that later).

That first sip at age 16 got me into the habit of drinking on the weekends. After a while, I had the idea in my head that if I wasn't going out and partying, I wasn't living life to the fullest.

When I studied abroad in Seville, I was in my sophomore and junior years of college. Spain had a completely different culture, and the drinking age was only 18 there. Alcohol was so cheap, and every night there seemed to be a celebration going on. The Spanish culture allowed for *botellones*, otherwise known as drinking parties, in big open plazas. On top of this, the clubs and bars didn't close until 7 a.m. There were always festivals and parties going on until the wee hours of the morning.

I remember doing crazy things when I drank alcohol. I would walk home on cobblestone streets with no shoes or socks on because my feet hurt from my boots. I would get into fights with people, and sometimes I would steal things. I would sleep in random places, and I would yell and be obnoxious. I was even robbed a couple of times because I wasn't paying attention in my drunken state.

Ever since 1847, Seville has celebrated a 7-day flamenco dancing festival every year called *La Feria de Abril*. The festival was 24/7, and it was a vacation week from school, so naturally, I took advantage. I went out and drank all night, every night, slept during the day, and then started the cycle over again. Looking back into my journal of my time studying in Spain, I found that I wrote, *I am drinking like an alcoholic!* Little did I know, I was one.

Alcohol got me into all kinds of trouble. It led me to be in abusive relationships, it led me to sleep with random men, and it led me to spend exorbitant amounts of money on my credit card that I didn't have. It caused me to have random fights with girls at bars, it gave me the courage to steal things from people, and it led me to be dishonest and hurt others who were close to me. Basically, it led me to have no boundaries at all, and it also showed how little love and self-care I had for myself. Soon living with no boundaries became the norm for me, and I was no longer a sweet and innocent little girl.

Alcohol also led me to a dark place. Alcoholism is a selfish, lonely disease. I isolated myself and shut out those that I loved. I missed important celebrations and family events because I preferred to party or was too drunk to show up. I quickly found myself drunk more often than not, but I would try to hide it from those who were closest to me. I am not proud to say that I would drive drunk often and endanger myself and others, but I did. At one point, I was basically living out of my dented car so that I didn't have to live with my parents and face them drunk every night.

Alcohol caused me to be loud, obnoxious, and overly emotional. It caused breakups, arguments, and depression. It caused me to be unclear about what I wanted, and it eventually led to my first divorce. Alcohol made me messy and embarrassing in front of others. It caused me to fall and fail. Yup, I was "that girl" that no one wanted to be around.

But to all this, I was blind. To me, I was living my life to the fullest. At least that is what I told myself. Alcohol equaled my best life. Everyone I knew partied hard, especially on the weekends, so it was normal, or so I thought.

By the age of 25, I was drinking hard core. I was going through a separation from my first husband, and I was working for an attorney as a paralegal in Boston. I remember the liquor store behind the law office in the parking lot. One day, I remember feeling really anxious, like I needed something to take the edge off. I found myself staring at the liquor store during work and thought about going to buy alcohol on my lunch break. The attorney was not in the office much, and some days she did not come in at all. *But what if she comes in and I get caught smelling like alcohol?* I thought.

Thankfully, I never ended up drinking during work for the four years that I worked there, but I was tempted numerous times. I am grateful to this day that I valued my job and the relationship that I had with the attorney more than I valued alcohol.

Instead of drinking at work, I decided to wait until it was time to go home. I went to the liquor store at 6 p.m. and drove home while simultaneously drinking four little bottles of Sutter Home wine. Being stuck for two hours in Boston traffic on the Massachusetts Turnpike was NOT a good time every evening, and so this soon became a habit.

I would fill up my water bottle with the four bottles of wine before I started my journey home and throw out the bottles so there was no evidence. Only by the grace of God did I make it home safe without injuring myself or others every single time. It is truly amazing that I never got a DUI. Even though I was pulled over drunk numerous times, I never got caught or tested for being drunk, even though I often was.

Walter was my first husband and was from Brazil. He was a good man, but we got married when I was 22 and he was 19. He couldn't even drink legally at our wedding. Why did I get married at 22? We didn't even know who we were as people at that young age! And, with his workaholic tendencies and my drinking, we found ourselves headed for divorce after 3 years of marriage. Shortly after the separation from Walter, I was out at a Brazilian live music venue with some friends when I met a second Brazilian guy named Marc.

I fell quick and hard for Marc, and physically I was super attracted to him. Our connection was insane, and we had so much fun together. The best part about Marc was that he was kind and generous. He would always buy me things and take me to dinner. He always had cash on him, and money was no object. We would drink and laugh and have a great time wherever we went.

Marc and I did a lot together. We went to concerts and went on a trip to Miami, Florida together, and we both had the same mentality around alcohol: that it equaled living life to the fullest.

Soon after we started dating, I noticed that when we would go to parties, Marc would frequently get into arguments or fights with other guys at the party. He became very jealous of me with his friends, even though there was nothing going on between us. We moved in together very quickly and got serious fast. We left the apartment he was living in with roommates and decided to live in an attic apartment together in a town just outside of Boston. We also decided to get a little Maltese dog named Jack.

I was sure that Marc was my soulmate at the time, and I was madly in love with him. But soon the drinking for both of us became very heavy, and Marc would get angry when he drank. Any little thing would set him off, and his personality would change in an instant. He would go from happy and joking around to angry and enraged, especially when he was drinking whiskey. He pushed me a few times, and threw things against the wall. But most of the time, I was also completely drunk and thought it was funny or nothing serious to be worried about.

One evening in December, he came home from work and asked to borrow my car to run to the store. I agreed and decided to make dinner for us while he went out. What I thought was going to be a quick run to the market turned into 3 hours. He had been gone for a while, and he wasn't picking up my calls. It seemed his phone had been shut off.

Many hours later, he returned home drunk out of his mind. He came home with a big jug of red wine and a 30-pack of beer. He was incredibly quiet and came over to where I was sitting on the sofa. He put the alcohol down and out of nowhere, he lunged at me. He also picked up Jack and threw him against the wall. He started hitting me and threw me to the ground. He got on top of me and claimed that he had heard that I was trying to get back together with my ex, Walter. This was of course a completely false accusation! I didn't even speak to Walter anymore. I tried to tell him, but he was too drunk to listen and didn't believe me.

That physical fight continued for about an hour. We were rolling around and punching, kicking, and pushing each other for what seemed like eternity. Marc worked out often and was a really strong man. At that moment, I was grateful that I had never been a small woman, which gave me a chance to fight back. The walls were paper thin, and I was praying that our neighbor downstairs would hear us fighting and would call the police, but that did not happen. I am sure he heard us, but he did not call the police.

At one point, Marc got on top of me with his hands around my neck. I thought to myself, *This might be it.*

With the little strength that I had left, I yelled out, "God help me!" and for some reason, Marc let go and stopped. I consider it a true miracle.

He laughed an evil laugh and got off of me. He said, "Get your stuff and get the fuck out of here, girl."

Was he really letting me go? I thought to myself. I didn't take any more time to think about it. I went into the bedroom and grabbed my laundry basket of clothes, Marc's passport, and $200 of his money on the dresser. He was too drunk to notice that I took it. When I went to get Jack, he was nowhere to be found, and Marc told me that he had let him go in the street and that he had run away.

My eyes filled up with tears, and I was not sure what I was more heartbroken about: my relationship or the dog. I did not have time to think about it and knew I just had to get out of there as soon as possible before Marc got angry again.

As I walked out the door, Marc started threatening me. He said that if I went to the police and they deported him, that he would come back to the US through Mexico and kill me, or hire someone else to kill me. With that bold statement, I slammed the door and ran down the stairs.

I started sobbing as soon as I got outside. The cold December air filled my lungs, and I felt like I couldn't breathe. Part of me was relieved that I had made it out of there alive, but I was so sad about the whole situation and could not believe what had just happened.

Devastated and exhausted, I carried my stuff to the car, and when I got there, Jack was sitting on the front seat! I was so happy to see him. Marc must have put him in the car when I was gathering my clothes and lied to me about it. Either way, I was ecstatic and hugged Jack for a minute as I cried, and he shook from the cold.

I pulled the car down the street, so I was away from the apartment, and pulled over next to a lake. I sobbed long and hard, and I had to figure out where I was going to go for the night. It was already dark, and I could barely see out of my left eye. Should I go to the police?

No, I was too scared of what would happen if Marc didn't get locked up and he came to find me. He said he would kill me. I could not go home and tell my parents looking a mess like I did. I didn't want them to see me like that. I also couldn't stop shaking. I decided to text my friend Leo to see if I could stay at his house. I asked if I could come over, and he agreed.

From the moment he opened the door, he knew something was wrong. I told him everything that had happened. I had marks and bruises all over my body, and so he helped me take photos of them. He strongly encouraged me to go to the police, but I shared with him my fear of Marc killing me if I went and they let him go and he came after me.

We ended up just talking most of the night and drinking. I wanted to numb myself and push down the pain and the reality of the situation that had just happened. I still couldn't believe it. It had all happened so fast. I wanted to wake up and have this all be a nightmare, but I knew it wasn't. It had happened. Yes, this had really happened.

The next day, I was going to have to face my parents, because I had nowhere else to go. I was almost as scared to tell my parents the truth as I was of Marc.

The next day, I woke up, and my body felt like it had been run over by a Mack truck. *Maybe I could get away with not telling my parents what happened, and I could just tell them we broke up?* I got up and looked in the mirror in the bathroom, and the bruises were inescapable. Purple, green, and yellow bruises and scratches covered my face, neck, and my body. My eye was purple and almost closed shut from the swelling. Crap, there was no way of hiding it; I was going to have to tell my parents.

I decided to call my mom as I was driving home from Leo's house. I told her everything that had happened, and when I arrived home, my dad opened the door with open arms. I just cried in his embrace as the night before flashed through my mind. It all still seemed like a dream, except the pain all over my body told me that it was not. I was truly lucky to be alive.

LESSONS LEARNED

Do not let anyone mistreat you... ever. You deserve to be treated like a queen with respect, love, and honor from any partner that you have. No relationship is worth being abused. If abuse happens once, it will happen again, and it will just get worse and worse due to its crazy cycle. Don't be afraid to leave any situation or relationship that is unhealthy. You are enough just the way you are. I promise it will be okay if you love yourself enough to leave.

CAPÍTULO CUATRO: THIRD TIME'S A CHARM

When we reached the end of Calle Betis, I saw The Phoenix Pub. *Oooooh the Phoenix,* I thought, and I let out a big sigh. "That is the bar that I used to meet all of my friends at to watch the soccer games," I told Anderson. "That is also the bar where I met Ahmed, my second husband," I explained. I felt a sense of heaviness inside immediately.

So, I am going to let that cat out of the bag. From the little that I have shared about myself, you may have put one and two together already, but yes, I have been married three times. Yup, you heard me right, THREE. Is it something I am proud of? No. Has each marriage taught me a valuable lesson, absolutely. I used to be super embarrassed to tell people, but I have an amazing relationship with my husband now, and I am the happiest I have ever been, so I am over it. It just took me three times to get here!

As I mentioned before, I first got married at the young age of 22 to Walter. Walter was 19 when he asked me to marry him, and we had only been together for a year before he asked me. I had met him one year prior at my welcome home party from Spain. My sister was dating his cousin at the time and had a party at his home to celebrate my return from studying abroad.

Walter was tall, dark, and handsome. He was light-hearted and fun, and we had similar interests. He was a really hard worker and always had two or three jobs. He worked so hard that he worked 80 hours a week, every week, which didn't leave much time for us. He was a good man, but my drinking had picked up during the time I spent alone while he was working. I felt lonely, and various events occurred on both sides of the relationship that led to its demise. He was a great guy, but just not the one for me.

The night that Walter and I went out to celebrate our one-year anniversary in the Italian North End of Boston, he was super quiet and hardly said a word at dinner. After dinner as we were ready to pull out of the parking lot, he nervously kneeled on top of me in the car and asked me to marry him. The strange statement that followed after he asked me to marry him was, "Let's get married and keep it a secret."

For those of you who don't know me personally, I like foreign men. After my first American boyfriend dumped me in college, I never dated another American again. I prefer the different language, exotic culture, and sexy accents that have always won me over. To me, Americans were boring, and this 19-year-old fiancé of mine was Brazilian and wanted to marry me! *Finally! My true love!* I thought, after he asked me.

From my experience with the Brazilian culture (Brazilians don't judge me!), oftentimes, one gets jealous of what the other one has. If someone saw Walter getting married to a young American woman, they might want to get married too. He claimed that the reason he asked me to keep it a secret was because my two sisters were also dating two Brazilians. One was Walter's cousin and the other one was his best friend. He feared that if they knew we were getting married, they would get jealous and try to convince my 18-year-old sisters to get married too.

And so, we kept it a secret from almost everybody. We told my parents and Walter's uncle, who attended the ceremony. We picked a muggy July summer day in 2005 and reserved a room at our favorite restaurant, found a Justice of the Peace, and tied the knot.

Only years later, after my sisters had ended things with the other two Brazilians, did I tell them about the marriage. As you can imagine, my sisters were hurt and upset that they were not included in the secret or the wedding. My fuzzy head from drinking often caused my actions to be fuzzy. We did end up having a huge wedding and celebration a year or so later with 250 people. Even though they were the bridesmaids, I can see why they would be hurt for not being included in the small ceremony the first time. I apologized to them years later for my hurtful actions.

I found myself questioning myself and wondering why I did not push back and tell Walter that it was important that they be included. Why couldn't I say no? Honestly, I did not expect the proposal on our one-year anniversary, and I was not ready. We hadn't even talked about marriage at that point. Looking back in hindsight, the chances of my sisters wanting to get married at that time if they found out were slim to none. I knew deep inside that it was not the right thing to do, but I did it anyway.

My second marriage was to a Moroccan man named Ahmed. Just seeing his name makes me cringe. After working for four years at the law firm in Boston, I decided to move back to Seville, Spain, and work as an English teacher. It was *Semana Santa* (Holy Week), which was kind of like spring break, and so I had the week off from school.

One of my roommates had just moved out of my apartment to go back to Germany. Before she left, she did not clean out her side of the refrigerator. When I went into the kitchen for dinner, I opened the fridge and noticed that she had left behind an unopened bottle of wine. *Oooooh!* I thought to myself. *How I would die for a glass of wine to start off this vacation and just relax!* At that point, I was about three and a half years into my sobriety.

I took the bottle out, put it on the counter, and just stared at it. I stared at it for a looong time. I stood there for a good 30 minutes and went back and forth in my mind as to whether I should open it and have a glass or not. The obsession with drinking had already returned, and I hadn't even put the wine to my lips yet.

I had recently gone through a tough breakup in December, a few months before, and had not really dealt with those feelings. I did not have any closure with the way that the relationship ended, being that he was in Boston and I was in Spain. After so many Alcoholics Anonymous meetings, you would think that I would have been ok, but the disease of Alcoholism is extraordinarily strong and sneaky. I thought to myself, *Just a glass or two won't hurt.*

And so I took out the bottle opener and began to open the wine. My heart was pounding, and I felt nervous and anxious as if I was committing a crime. As I poured the red wine into a glass and took a sip, I felt a sudden relief run down my body, like all my cares had gone away. The dryness of the wine resonated on my tongue, and I felt like I had found my long-lost friend.

In AA, they say, "The first drink is the worst drink and is the one that gets you drunk." This basically translates into, "Once you start, you cannot stop." And that could not have been truer for me.

I quickly finished the whole bottle of wine, and I found myself leaving my house at 10 o'clock at night to try to find a store that was open for me to buy another bottle. It was late, and most of the grocery stores were closed, especially because of the Easter holiday. But that strong desire to have more had returned instantly, and so I needed to find a place that was open. I walked across the bridge into town to the convenience store that I knew sold alcohol a little later. It was more expensive there, but I didn't care. At that point, I just needed more.

After the first night of breaking my sobriety, I had drunk 3 bottles of wine by myself, and had smoked a whole pack of cigarettes. I had just started smoking again days before I drank the wine. Cigarettes and alcohol in Spain were unbelievably cheap, and the two had always gone hand in hand for me. Once I started smoking, I should have known that drinking was right around the corner.

The drinking in my apartment continued for five days straight. The whole vacation week was gloomy and rainy, and so I had no real reason to leave my apartment. Each day, I would go out to the store and stock up on wine and snacks and go home and lock myself in my room. I would smoke the cigarettes and drink the wine until I threw up. Each morning, I would wake up feeling horrible, and I would get on my knees and ask God to remove the obsession of drinking.

On the fifth day of drinking, I woke up, and something inside me had changed. I had planned an excursion with some friends to Aracena, a small town outside of Seville filled with cute white houses and was known for its amazing organic *jamón serrano* (Spanish ham). Because of the day trip with my friends, I had to get up and shower and get dressed. As I walked to the bathroom, I noticed I suddenly did not have the desire to drink anymore, so I went with them to Aracena.

When I got home that same day, I decided to go out to The Phoenix Pub to meet my girlfriends to watch the Barcelona soccer game. Thankfully, I didn't feel like drinking, and I just ordered a Coca Cola Light. After the game, as I was leaving to walk home, I passed in front of a guy who was standing at the door.

He said, "Hola!" I ignored him and continued walking down the main street towards my house.

As I was waiting at the traffic light to cross, the same man who had said hello to me popped out of nowhere and started talking to me. I hadn't realized it, but he had followed me out when I left the bar. My head and my heart were unclear at the time from the five days of drinking, and I never should have pursued anything with him. But that is what drinking does to an alcoholic. It takes away all clarity and turns you into a person that you do not want to be.

The man who followed me home seemed like a gentleman. His name was Ahmed, and he was originally from Morocco. He was a student in Seville who had arrived around the same time that I did.

I told him I was not looking for a boyfriend, but he was very persistent to take me out. It seemed like getting me to date him was almost like a game. Even after I told him that I did not want a relationship, he would not back down and would not take "no" for an answer. That was my first red flag right there, but after the breakup with my ex four months before, it was nice to feel wanted and desired again.

Another reason that I liked hanging around Ahmed is because he did not drink alcohol because he was Muslim. After just having my relapse with alcohol, I thought that I was safe dating him and that having him around could at least help me stay sober for a while. I really did not want to drink again.

Soon my "no" to Ahmed turned into months of dating. Ahmed was serious, rugged, and tough, but he also had a warm compassionate side to him too. After I told him about my relapse with alcohol, Ahmed thought that it was best if I did not go out late at night with my friends anymore because it wasn't a good idea to be around alcohol.

I suppose he is right about that, I thought, and before I had realized it, I had cut off all contact with my friends. Soon, the only person I was really hanging out with in Seville outside of my job was Ahmed.

Ahmed and I argued A LOT. Most of the arguments were over differences in our perceptions of situations that we did not see eye to eye on. Sometimes it was related to our religious beliefs since I grew up Catholic and he was Muslim. Other times it was about societal issues, the way I dressed, my interaction with men, talking with guys who were coworkers, family members, friends and the list of issues went on. Ahmed and I were both passionate people, and so any fight that we felt strongly about often led to yelling and screaming.

At one point, I started to question myself and our relationship. I started to feel like Ahmed was trying to control me. I didn't like being told what to do, who to hang out with, where to go, how to dress, or what religion I "should" be. So, naturally, I would fight back. I had always considered myself a pretty independent woman and did not like the fact that he was trying to control my every move. He had a cunning way of manipulating me and making me think that the decisions I made were my ideas when, really, they were his that he was trying to push on me.

About a year into our relationship, my sisters came to visit us for the holiday week, which was during the *Feria de Abril*. They were really excited to get to know him, but things did not turn out the way we had planned. He ended up being quite rude to them, and we got into numerous arguments while they were visiting. I still had to go to teach English when they were visiting, and he had agreed to help out and take them around the city while I was at work. He ended up abandoning them, saying that he didn't speak enough English to hang out with them and left them on their own. My sisters did not speak any

Spanish, but they managed their way around the city by themselves.

One of the last nights that my sisters were in town, we went to dinner without Ahmed. During dinner, they expressed their concern for my relationship with him. They didn't feel like he was right for me and were worried about how much we fought. They saw that I was unhappy, which, to be honest, I was. Because of the fighting and the control that he tried to have, I wasn't much of a host to them. I was either arguing with Ahmed, meeting him to try to smooth things over, or coming home early so he would not get mad at me again for being out late and accusing me of being with other man, or some crazy accusation like that.

But of course, blind and in love, I didn't listen to them. I thought, They don't know the REAL Ahmed. He takes care of me and really loves me.

The second year that Ahmed and I were together, we moved into an apartment in the center of Seville. Ahmed proposed to me on my 30th birthday trip to Paris next to the Eiffel Tower. Although I was ecstatic, I knew deep down inside that something wasn't right with our relationship. Ironically, he also got me a ring that I hated. There was a fake diamond in the middle with fake diamonds surrounding it on the sides that were in a setting that I thought was hideous. That should have been a clue right there! If he really knew me well, he would have known that I hated the ring he gave me.

Naturally, when I told him how I really felt about the ring, he got angry. It took a couple of tries, but we finally found one that was a good fit for me. I am not materialistic at all, but I thought if I was going to wear the ring for the rest of my life, I better like it.

While we were in Paris, he met my best friend Mik who had flown all the way from Boston to be with us on my 30th birthday.

He naturally didn't like Mik because he was a man, and he knew me better than anyone else. Ahmed saw how close we were, and he was immediately jealous. But again, that didn't stop me from getting engaged to him.

The following summer, we decided that we were going to apply for a fiancé k-1 visa for Ahmed, move back to the United States, and get married. I was torn about the decision because I loved Spain so much. When I moved there two years previously, I had not planned to go back to live in the USA, at least not so soon. But Ahmed had been out of work for almost two years in Spain. I saw how depressed he was, and with the economic crises in Spain, there was no way that he was going to find a job. With just my teacher salary, I could not make enough money for both of us to live on and have a future there. So we decided it was best to move back to Boston, get married, and get Ahmed working papers in the US so we could have a future.

The process to get a fiancé visa was very arduous, but we managed to do it. Paper after paper, document after document, an all-day interview in Madrid, financial sponsorship from my parents, documents translated, photos to show our relationship, and handing over our passports, Ahmed was finally awarded the fiancé visa.

I decided to move home first so I could start planning our wedding. As usual, when I left Sevilla on the plane, my eyes filled with tears. Doubts filled my head, and I wondered if I was making the right decision. Aside from that, Ahmed wanted to go home to Morocco to say good-bye to his family one last time before moving to America. The period apart was very stressful, and we argued often when we were apart.

Ahmed would get frustrated because he was stuck in Spain with no job waiting for his passport to be returned to him from the embassy. To make matters worse, I was far away from him without being under his control. There were many times that I thought about calling off the marriage because the arguments got so bad. But I kept telling myself that he was just frustrated with the current situation and it would get better once we were together again.

I remember one time he was mad about something and kept calling my parent's house phone because I wouldn't answer my cell phone. My dad answered to tell him to stop calling the house repetitively and asked him to give me some space.

But still, I ignored all the signs and went through with the wedding. We had already put a large deposit down, and I kept telling myself that Ahmed was acting this way because he was sad, depressed, and away from me.

I look back now and ask myself, *How could I keep telling myself these lies? How could I believe them and be so blind?* But that was just where I was in my life, and I think I wanted the fairytale ending of falling in love in my favorite city in the world and living happily ever after.

It wasn't a surprise when Ahmed arrived in the USA and the fighting continued. I kept telling myself that everything was new for him. He was going through a culture shock. The weather was cold. He didn't have a job yet, or his working papers, a car, a license, friends, or know where anything was. He didn't speak English, and we were stuck at my parents' house in a small town outside of Boston for the first couple of months. Again, I kept telling myself that it was all a culture shock, and once he got settled, learned the language, and adapted, everything would be ok.

But everything was not okay. I can tell you story after story of fight after fight and issue after issue with Ahmed. No matter what I did, I was always the one to blame, and I was never good enough for him no matter how hard I tried. Things would get really bad between us, but then we would make up and they would get really good for a while. I would avoid issues that were a sore subject so that we wouldn't start fighting, and every day was like walking on eggshells around him. And then something would make him upset, the cycle would start its course again, and things would get really bad.

I started seeing a counselor for marriage problems and depression 6 months after Ahmed and I got married. We also tried seeing a counselor in Spanish together. The first meeting with her, he walked out on both of us and said the relationship was over, but by the time I got home, he was sad, sorry, and ready to make up again. Everything was a game with him and so up and down. I constantly questioned myself, my values, and my actions, because Ahmed made me feel horrible and always blamed me for things that in his eyes were "wrong." He would treat me poorly and use private information that I shared with him or personal struggles or stories against me when he got angry. Then he would go after my family and friends and bring them into the fights too. I got really tired of the fighting, but I did not want to get divorced again, so I stayed.

Various times in our relationship situations caused me to stay at friends' houses or escape to a hotel for a night or two where I could feel at peace and safe and gather my thoughts. At one point, I moved out of our apartment in Boston. A friend of mine from AA let me rent a room from her and stay at her peaceful home hidden from him in a quiet neighborhood. I wanted Ahmed to know that I was serious and that if his behavior did not change, I would move out forever and he would lose me. Eventually I gave him another chance and I moved back in. It didn't take long before he was blaming me for something, threatening to throw me out on the street, locking me in our second bedroom, and mistreating me again. The relationship became so mentally and physically exhausting, and so many times I felt helpless.

The last straw came in May of 2016. One weeknight around 11 p.m., my sister called me to tell me that she had found a second Facebook page that was Ahmed's. I went to my phone to look at it, and all of his friends on the page were Latina women from Boston wearing sexy clothes, or almost naked. I was absolutely shocked. I could NOT believe my eyes. After everything I did for him and all that I had put up with from him, he had the nerve to have a secret page and try to hide it from me? He could have at least been smart and made the page private... but he didn't. It was almost like he wanted me to find it.

I immediately had flashbacks to all the times that he got upset because he thought I was looking at another guy or had a friend on Facebook who was a guy. God forbid I even looked in the direction of a man; he would flip out and get angry. And that was all the truth that I needed to end things with him. I had had enough of the mistreatment, the hypocrisy, the manipulation, and the abuse. My heart was worn and deflated, and I could not take anymore.

Ahmed heard me on the phone with my sister and came next to me to listen. Once he realized what she was telling me, he demanded that I hang up the phone and not listen to her. He kept saying that it was none of her business and asked why she was telling me these things.

When I hung up the phone, my sister was clearly concerned for my safety. I tried speaking to him in a calm manner and demanded that he show me the page. He refused at first, but then I threatened to call my parents and tell them, so he showed me. It turns out that he had created the page about 8-months prior, right after our wedding anniversary in October when things were GOOD with us! I could not believe it! I was truly flabbergasted. He rarely used the page and only commented a few things on the girls' profiles, but still, the fact that he had created it and he was a married man was just wrong.

I was done with the disrespect, done with the verbal threats, done with the emotional and mental abuse, and done with all the fighting. I was outraged and so hurt, and of course, we started arguing. He couldn't even take responsibility for it, and he kept blaming my sister! I tried to compare the situation and asked what he would do if this happened to his sister, but there was no point of even trying to reason with him. He would never see it my way or admit to doing anything wrong, which made me even more frustrated.

I told him I was going to sleep on the coach in the second bedroom, and he said, "No way!" "Married women sleep with their husbands in the same bed."

And I said, "Married men don't have secret Facebook pages with other women!"

And so the fight went. The fight went on for hours. It got so heated, and before I knew it, he physically lunged at me. I put my leg up and my arms toward his chest to block him and defend myself, and I whacked him. He immediately stepped back and yelled at me and said that I had attacked HIM and that I was abusing him. I could not believe that he lunged at me and then had the nerve to blame it on me. It was complete insanity.

And that, right there, is a summary of what he did our entire relationship. Everything he did, he twisted around and tried to point it at me. So much so, that I would question myself over and over again, until I started to believe his lies were the truth. I even found myself questioning if I had lunged at him first, because he insisted that I had.

I knew the moment that he lunged at me that the relationship was truly over forever. There was no way that I could continue being married to a man that had 1) just physically attacked me, and 2) physically attacked me after discovering a Facebook page of women that HE had created. I deserved better for myself, and I knew that things would physically only become more dangerous going forward if I stayed. If he attacked me once, he would do it again.

Unfortunately, I knew from my experience with Marc that abusive relationships just get worse and eventually can become life-threatening. This meant that I had to find a way to leave. I felt soooooooo sad. I felt like he had just died right in front of me. I am sure he just suspected that this would be another one of our fights and that I would forgive him in a couple of days, but this time it was different. He did not know it was over, but I did. The worst part is, he would not "let me" move out. He, of course, had to be in control at all times, so whatever I wanted, he would not "allow me" to do, and he would demand that I do the opposite. I felt like a slave.

I scheduled a time to meet with my counselor. After explaining the incident, we decided together that I would wait a month for him to go on vacation back to his home in Morocco so that I could leave in a safe way on my own terms. Ahmed did not work in the summer since his job was to work on a school year schedule from September to May. The plan was for Ahmed to go first and I would go and meet him and his family in Morocco a couple of weeks later to visit. From there, we were going to travel on through Europe.

However, I secretly planned to leave him instead. Ahmed didn't even know it, but I was able to take a family leave period from my job for 5 days because of how depressed I was. During those five days while he was at work, I found a second apartment across the city. My parents lent me money for a deposit on the new apartment so he would not see anything come out of our bank account. I opened a separate bank account only in my name and a private P.O. Box for my mail so he wouldn't be able to find me.

During that month, I was forced to act "normal" until he left for his trip, and it was torture. It was so hard to be fake and pretend to be happy, but if he found out my plan, he wouldn't go to Morocco and he would do everything to stop it. Keeping this big secret from him was so hard, but I managed because I knew my life and my sanity were on the line.

The day I brought him to the airport, he could sense something was wrong. My eyes filled up with tears, because I knew it was really over, and that was going to be the last time that I would see him. Being the narcissist that he was, he naturally thought that I was just sad that he was leaving, but I knew inside that this was the end for us. As he walked away to the TSA security line, he turned around and looked back, and I waved good-bye.

As I walked out of the airport, my chest felt tight, and I started to breathe really heavily. I couldn't hold the tears back anymore. The reality of the end had hit me in the face, and the events of the last month replayed in my head. I felt sad and relieved all at the same time. I remember calling my friend, Jan, who had been such a source of support through all of this. I couldn't believe that this was my life and that my marriage had failed… again.

That same day, I packed everything up and moved all my things out into my new apartment. I wanted to get out of our apartment and leave behind all those horrible memories as soon as possible. My dad came over to help me. Sadly, this was not the first time that he was helping me move to escape an abusive relationship.

Why do I attract these crazy abusive men? I thought. I am going to have to work on myself to change that.

Most of the things we owned were wedding gifts. I didn't want the memories anyway, so I left them in the apartment for Ahmed when he returned. The day I was supposed to leave to travel to Morocco to meet him, I took out exactly half of the money in our savings account and deposited it in my new bank account. Then I paid the next month's rent and called the landlord to tell him that I was moving out and that any rent going forward would be coming from Ahmed.

I immediately was filled with relief and deep sadness at the same time. Memories, good and bad, flooded my mind. Marriage number 2 was over. How could it be that I was going to be divorced AGAIN at age 33?! Some people don't even get married until they are 33! I had a lot of work to do on myself. I was really left scarred and depleted from this one.

Eventually, with time, things got better. As you can imagine, Ahmed did not take the news very well, and he flipped out when he received the notification that half of the savings had been removed from the bank account. Things got worse for me before they got better, but I know for a fact that I would not be where I am today without everything that happened. I probably would not be alive to tell the story.

Leaving that abusive relationship was the best thing that I ever did for myself. It taught me a lot about my strength, my grace and about relationships. After I got over the initial stage of sadness, I had hope. It gave me purpose. I returned to the old Christine who was happy and free to do anything she wanted again without having to tiptoe around him or get permission. The whole world was in front of me and open again with new possibilities.

Instead of meeting Ahmed in Morocco and traveling with him, I went on a trip to Europe with my dad for two weeks. We quickly planned a trip to different places than Ahmed and I had planned to go to and had an amazing time. We went to Sweden, Denmark, Finland, and Russia, and when my dad left me to go back to work, I continued on by myself to Estonia and Greece. I was so grateful that my dad was there to support me and to be a shoulder to cry on during that difficult time. I will forever cherish those memories and the time we spent together.

LESSONS LEARNED

Love is blind. If you see signs of abuse, find a safe way to leave because the relationship will only get worse. No relationship is worth risking your life or your sanity over. You are enough the way you are, and don't let anyone tell you or make you think otherwise. Love yourself by putting your safety and sanity first and by having the courage to leave the relationship if you feel you are in danger.

CAPÍTULO CINCO: VIP

As Anderson and I walked over the bridge and through the Maria Luisa park, I stared at the *Plaza de España* in awe at how majestic it was. No matter how many times I see it, there is still a sense of wonder that comes over me every time that I look up at the gigantic structure. As I stood there under the beaming sun and stared at all its brilliant colors, I bumped into a small, dark haired woman who rudely grunted, *"Ten cuidado chica!"* (Watch out, girl!) and walked away.

Running into this woman reminded me of Michaela, the woman I used to work for who owns VIP Management in Miami, Florida. I was hired by her as a project manager right before I moved to Miami and was so excited to work with her company. Although the hiring process was quite gruesome with many different interviews between her and her VP, she had been super warm and helpful from the beginning by offering information that was valuable as a new resident of Miami. Even before I was hired, she would often text me and send me photos of my new neighborhood and the beach to get me excited. When I arrived in Florida, she seemed to go out of her way to recommend anything that Anderson and I needed. This included a reputable hair salon, introducing me to people, a place to fix our car, restaurants to try, hurricane tips, and whatever else we needed.

Michaela had gone through a tough divorce with an alcoholic who still lived in the area. Once I felt comfortable with her, I opened up with her about my experience with alcohol, and also my past relationship with another alcoholic, and we seemed to bond over these common experiences. She had a lot of questions, and not being an alcoholic herself, she never understood the disease, so I was happy to share my experiences with it to help her understand.

My job for Michaela was to manage other members of the team who worked for her. I had to make sure projects were completed on time and edited and reviewed correctly for the client (or so I thought). I was new to the area of management, which she knew when I was hired, and there were new systems and tools for me to learn in order to get up to speed and be able to do my job efficiently. When she hired me, she persuaded me to agree to work for $5 an hour less than my rate with my other clients because I lacked experience. I accepted it because I saw the opportunity for growth and I was looking for stable clients with enough hours to keep a steady income, so I agreed.

After a couple of weeks of working there, things started to change. I soon learned that Michaela was super controlling, and everything had to be done exactly the way she wanted. Everything was fake about Michaela: her tan, her breasts, her teeth, and her personality. Even though I had 5 other virtual assistant clients that I was working with, she demanded that I work from her house from about 10 a.m. to 6 p.m., which didn't leave me much free time to do other client work.

Michaela was very strong-willed and controlling. It didn't take long for me to be afraid to tell her if I had work to do for my other clients. Instead, I would have to get up super early and do the work before I went to her house or wait until 5 or 6 p.m. when I went home to complete it. I often would get annoyed because I would go to her house when she asked at 10, and then she would remain on the phone for thirty to sixty minutes after I arrived with me just sitting there twiddling my thumbs. This was a lack of respect of my time and also time that I could be working on projects for my other clients.

Michaela would work for hours straight without taking a break. Let me rephrase, without taking a *healthy* break. What I mean by this is that she smoked cigarettes, and she smoked them often inside of her apartment. Each day, I would go to her home for work and leave the building feeling gross and smelling of cigarette smoke. I told her in the beginning that I did not like smoking and that I had asthma, but I guess she did not care. She thought that smoking the cigarettes far away from me off of her balcony in a studio apartment did not affect me.

I remember talking on the phone with my sister one day, and she asked me, "What is up with your voice? You sound different."

My voice was vividly changing due to being around cigarettes each day, and I started to develop a cough. I began to feel very unhappy and stressed, and often I even went home with migraines.

After the first couple of weeks, Michaela's personality had changed too. A boss lady who was once a nice, helpful woman turned into a witch who ordered me to do her bitch work and errands. I don't know why, but she did not trust me with the system that we used to keep track of the work that we did. I was constantly anxious when I was with her, and the pressure that I felt with her leaning over my shoulder caused me to make mistakes sometimes. She would also have me make these annoying phone calls, tell me what to say, and even have me lie so she would get what she wanted. I was so nervous with her sitting right there staring at me that I would forget what I was supposed to say, and then she would get mad and tell me to hang up. If I did make a mistake, she would scold me, and I would feel ashamed.

Then the personal tasks started. I soon found myself at the mall returning clothes for her, bringing her car to get fixed, buying things for her, getting her coffee, and other crazy errands. I thought to myself, *This is not what I signed up for. What happened to being a project manager?* On one hand, I was happy to be out of her smoky apartment, but on the other hand, I was not hired to be running errands all day.

The last straw came when she asked me to go to Walgreens and return a set of makeup bags. It bothered me because I saw that she had already used them and had cleaned the makeup out of them to make it look like they were new. Walgreens return policy was 30 days with the receipt in order to get the cash back, and it had been about 40 days since she had bought them, which meant that it was past the allowed return time.

The first time I went to return the makeup bags, the cashier told me that I could not return them because the 30 days return period had passed. I called Michaela to let her know, and she told me to speak with the supervisor. They called the supervisor over, and she explained the same thing to me, but said I could exchange the bags for another item in Walgreens. When I told this to Michaela, she told me to buy $40 of cigarettes in exchange for the bags. When I tried to purchase the cigarettes, the supervisor said that I could not purchase cigarettes or milk with store credit, that it was the store policy and not allowed. She even showed me that the register would physically not complete the transaction.

When I called Michaela to tell her this, she was extremely frustrated and demanded to speak to the supervisor herself. After berating the supervisor on duty on speaker phone, she gave us the store manager's phone number and said we could call him the next day to see if there was anything he could do. Michaela was not happy with me or the store, and I went home that night feeling worn out, angry, frustrated, used, dirty from cigarette smoke, and undervalued.

Is this what I left my job as a project manager at Harvard for? I thought to myself. I am not one to brag or think super highly of myself, but I thought, I have a master's degree from Harvard University, and I am sitting here arguing about exchanging cigarettes for used makeup bags at Walgreens.

It just did not feel right. Thinking of the silliness of the entire situation at the moment, I burst out laughing. It was silly, but it was also serious and true. This was the reality that my life had come to.

I decided it wasn't right, but I also knew that if I was going to get out of this job, I was going to have to face Michaela and tell her. She had spent a lot of time training me on her company systems and had also helped me get established in Miami, and I felt guilty. She also took me to lunch every day, which I enjoyed, and we would talk about life and men and fun things. However, none of these things were worth feeling miserable for a job that I was doing that I hated. I felt like I was tricked. This was not what I had signed up for when I was hired.

After crying numerous nights from being unhappy and speaking with Anderson, I decided that I had to end this working relationship. Anderson reminded me that I ran my own company and that I was the BOSS, not Michaela. SHE was MY client. I was not being valued, and I was not using the skills I had to do work that fulfilled me. There is nothing wrong with being a personal assistant, but I had done that many years ago and that was not what I wanted to be doing in my business. I just had to figure out how I was going to tell Michaela that I was leaving her.

I dreaded returning to work the next day. I knew she was going to have me call the Walgreens store manager, or even go back in person to try to negotiate the exchange for cigarettes. When I arrived at her home, she asked me to return a skirt at H

& M that did not fit her and exchange it for a different skirt. She asked me to call the Walgreens store manager on the way to the mall. *Yayyy,* I thought, *my two favorite things to do!* as I walked out the door and rolled my eyes.

As in the past, she gave me instructions on EXACTLY what I should say to the store manager. Her excuse for not returning the bags at an earlier date was because she had gone to the West Coast of Florida to help with the devastation of Hurricane Michael. While this was true, she was gone for only a few days, and not an entire 2 weeks like she instructed me to say. Again, she was asking me to lie for her just to get what she wanted from Walgreens.

As I drove towards the mall to return the skirt, I contemplated lying and telling her that I called the Walgreens manager and he said no because I knew that was what he was going to say anyway. After thinking about the lie, I thought that I should call, even though it was uncomfortable because that was not who I was. I was an honest person.

So I gave the manager a call. As suspected, even after saying that she had gone to help with the hurricane cleanup, he said that the store physically could not exchange the bags for cigarettes in their system and that the store credit would have to be used for something else instead of cigarettes. I dreaded telling Michaela and decided I would return the skirt first and tell her when I got back.

When I arrived at H & M, there was a huge line of people. Michaela had asked me to get a different size, and so I waited patiently in the line to exchange it. When I returned to her home, I told her about the store manager, and she rolled her eyes and huffed and puffed out of frustration. When I gave her the new skirt, she looked at the receipt, and her face changed.

She looked at me and said, "What's up with this?" as she pointed to the receipt. She told me that the cashier had made a mistake and instead of exchanging the skirt, she had added another skirt to the receipt and charged her again. She said, "You're just going to have to go back and have her fix it."

At that moment, without even thinking, my immediate reaction was that I rolled my eyes and let out a big sigh of frustration. I had had it with running errands, her attitude, and her lies.

She said, "What's the matter, Christine?"

I had had enough. I could not take working with this woman any longer. It all came flooding out of me. I told her that I was having a hard time working with her, and I thought that I was hired to be a project manager, but really all I was doing was being her personal assistant. I told her I didn't think that she valued my skills and did not allow me to use the systems she had taught me because she was too controlling. I told her I did not enjoy running errands for her and that the cigarettes were really bothering me. We had an hour-long discussion, and I told her that I needed to go home and think long and hard about whether or not I wanted to continue working with her.

I left there with a migraine yet again and decided to walk home the three miles to my house that night to think about everything that had happened. It was all running through my head over and over and again.

This is not good, I thought. This is not healthy for me. I am not being valued for who I am and what I have to offer. I am inhaling cigarette smoke every day to the point that my voice is changing.

I decided I would sleep on it, and if I still felt the same way the next day, I would call Michaela and tell her that I was done. When I woke up the next morning, I still felt the same way. Actually, I felt worse and had a big pit in my stomach. It was Saturday, so I waited a few hours until the afternoon. I did not feel better, and the whole situation was consuming my mind and causing anxiety, so I decided to call her. I had a feeling that she was not going to answer the phone, and I was right. When I called her, it just rang and rang. She was probably on the other line talking about me to another one of her contractors as I had seen her do in the past with other situations that had happened. I left her a voicemail and asked her to call me back that afternoon because I had something important to speak with her about.

I was filled with anxiety the whole day about telling her that I was done working for VIP Management, but she never called me back. *So much for a relaxing Saturday,* I thought. I had seen her play this game with other contractors of hers, and I had a feeling that she would treat me the same way. So at 11:30 p.m., I sent my resignation email that I had prepared earlier in the day when I suspected that she wouldn't call me back. I also sent one to her VP of Operations.

I did not want to give my resignation that way, but I knew if I waited for her to call me back, I would not sleep all night. I was not prepared to have any more sleepless nights over this company or this woman.

I am glad that I did not wait for her to return my call, because it took her three days to call me back, even after I sent the email. That was her way of "having control" with her employees, and I was done playing her games. It was the best professional decision I ever made. Things ended up working out as I found a new client that replaced the income I was making at VIP with a client that I enjoyed working with a lot more.

LESSONS LEARNED

It is okay to say no, and it is okay to leave an unhealthy work environment. No amount of money or job is worth feeling anxious every single day. Life is too short to not do work that you love, so if it isn't a fit, it is okay to move on to something else without feeling guilty. You are enough and deserve happiness. Always listen to your gut, because it knows best. And love yourself.

CAPÍTULO SEIS: JUST SAY NO TO EGYPT

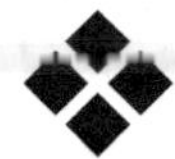

Walking though the *Plaza de España* with Anderson brought back so many memories. I remembered dates that I had gone on there, time with my family when they came to visit me, early morning runs that I went on through the park, walks, sunbathing with friends, and spontaneous flamenco dancers in the center of the plaza. As we walked by the vendors that had their items laid out on different colored blankets, it brought me back to my trip to Egypt and all the markets and vendors that I had to run away from there.

As I sat on my 10-hour fight from Egypt back to Miami, my mind was continuously trying to make sense of the trip that I had just gone on. What. Just. Happened? Was Egypt a real country? Do people really live that way? My mind was battling between trying to process all the things that had just happened while at the same time trying to block them out because I didn't want to remember.

I met my best friend Mik in Cairo, Egypt, where we traveled to various cities throughout the country, and then headed on to Tunisia and Milan to visit Mik's family. Words cannot describe the experiences that we had in Egypt, or how those experiences have changed us. I felt like I had been put through emotional torture. I felt violated. I felt dirty, used, and disrespected. I felt overwhelmed and taken advantage of. I was in disbelief that a culture could truly live the way that we had just experienced, but they do.

"Taxi? Horse ride? Where are you from? Let me show you something. Come take a look. Boat ride? Pay whatever makes you happy. You get a Ramadan discount. Everything is free! Maybe later? Just take a look. Where are you going? How can I help? Want a tour? Can I bring you somewhere? Do you want water? Are you from Germany? You must be Italian?"

These were just a few of the phrases that were constantly yelled out at us or in our faces the second we stepped outside of our hotel... or anywhere we went, for that matter. Not even off of the hotel property, Egyptian men began yelling these phrases from across the street. Forget trying to WALK down the street to an ATM, because when they pulled up beside you on their horse and buggy, they just followed you walking on the sidewalk and wouldn't leave you alone until you were forced to scream a rude strong "NO!!!" at them.

Mik and I were blown away at how disrespectful these men were to us day in and day out. Every single man that we encountered had an agenda to suck as much money and energy as they could from us. And when you gave them a little money, they always wanted more. I say "men," because it was rare to see a woman working, selling, driving, or interacting with tourists anywhere in Egypt. The only place we felt "safe" and unbothered was inside of the hotel. Could this be real? Were we stuck inside of a nightmare and just about to wake up? Could this be happening at one of the Seven Wonders of the World? Surely people could not live like this every day, but we quickly discovered they do.

Our first day was spent at the Pyramids in Giza. There is no arguing that they are an amazing site to see. As we dodged through the late-night Ramadan Cairo traffic, which consisted of animals, carts, motorcycles, scooters, buses with people hanging off of them, cars, and horses and buggies, we arrived at our hotel right outside the entrance to the pyramids. We were so excited to wake up and see the beautiful view of the sun rising over them. Little did we know what we were in for the next day.

After a tough negotiation session with the hotel concierge, we finally set on a price for a driver to take us to the pyramids, drop us off, and pick us up a few hours later. As we gazed at the pyramids as we got closer, the driver warned us about people giving us different prices for different things and told us that the general entrance ticket would get us in to see the pyramids and enter them all with the exception of the Great Pyramid located behind the entrance. We were also warned and had read in the guidebook that we would try to be charged a second time for entering certain pyramids, which didn't make us feel great.

After we bought our tickets, a man approached us telling us that he was a pyramid guide and showed us his badge. We hadn't even entered the site yet, and we were starting to get harassed.

As we kindly declined his services, he continued to follow us and yelled in a threatening voice, "Hey, hey! Come back here! Where are you from? I work here. Come here!"

As our brisk walk picked up to a slow jog, we found the entrance and went in. "Yikes!" we said. This was not a good start to seeing one of the Seven Wonders of the World. As you may imagine, the situation just got worse and worse as we ventured inside.

First, there was the guy who wanted us to pay him to take our photos with our own iPhones. He also showed us his badge that he worked there. Then there were dozens of guys on camels lurking around wanting to take us for a ride or take our photos on the camels. Then there were the emaciated horses attached to buggies who wanted to bring us for a ride around the vast pyramid area. Next there were the vendors trying to sell us souvenirs, wooden objects, postcards, water, and whatever other trinkets they could come up with. Then there were the guides who wanted to tell you all about the history of the pyramids in exchange for some exorbitant price.

Everywhere we went we were dodging vendors like bullets, having to decline with a harsh "NO!" every single time. They were so persistent and wouldn't take "no" for an answer, and they wanted you to bargain with them. Then you had the men who just walked around and wanted to tell you some facts about the pyramids in exchange for a tip. And when you gave them a tip, whatever you gave them was never enough. We quickly learned that it was best to just not engage at all, if you could somehow avoid them.

No matter how many times we said, "No, no, thank you, not today, maybe later, I am not interested..." they did not take any rejection for an answer. It reminded me of one of my bad relationships that I couldn't get out of no matter how hard I tried. I felt like I was dating Ahmed again! We just wanted to see the pyramids and marvel at their unique beauty without being bothered. Unfortunately, that was too much to ask for. Everywhere we went, we were endlessly hassled.

We attempted to enter one of the pyramids, and just as we had been warned when we showed our ticket, the men at the entrance demanded that we buy a second ticket. Not only did they tell us that we had to buy another ticket, but we had to do it back at the entrance, which was far away. With the 100-degree heat and our patience wearing thin, we decided to move on to another pyramid.

Then we decided that we would find one guy and try to just take some photos on his camel in front of the pyramids, because, hey, we were at the Egyptian Pyramids! We couldn't go home without a camel photo!

Boy, was that a mistake! We made it clear that we did not want a ride, and just wanted some photos. Before mounting the camel, I asked the man how much it was. His response was, "Whatever makes you happy, my dear."

At this point, we knew better than that, so I asked again. He repeated, "Whatever you can give me, I accept, my dear."

So Mik got on the camel, and then I followed. We probably took photos for about 15- 20 minutes total. At the end, we thanked the man, and Mik gave him Egyptian pounds, which were equivalent to $20 US Dollars. The man's face looked like we had only given him a dollar, and so the fun began…

The man came up to us and started complaining and asking for more, saying that he had done so much for us. I couldn't believe it. I wish I made $20 for 15 minutes of work! What made me even more mad was that he was using Ramadan as an excuse of why we should give him more money.

When I gave him $10 more (again, in his own currency), he STILL was not satisfied. I could feel my blood boiling, and it wasn't due to the 100-degree heat. I started arguing with the man, and Mik got the argument on video. Looking back at the video, the camel just stood there with a smirk on his face as if the situation was all too familiar to him. Something told me the camel had heard this conversation before. Needless to say, I did not give the man any more money.

It is unfortunate, but the trip just continued with stories similar to what happened at the pyramids. We started telling people we were from Canada when we were asked because we discovered they thought Americans had so much money. We stopped at a rest stop to use the bathroom for which I had to pay. The man at the rest stop became very angry because we did not want to go in and look at his store, and he spit in our direction and yelled, "All Canadians are bad!"

Another example was when we hired a driver who we thought we could trust who had taken us around the city of Luxor for the day. At the end of the day, we asked him to give us a price to do a day trip to Aswan, a Nubian city in the south of Egypt. We almost got scammed from him as he told us the price was $600. When we called our hotel to ask, they gave us a driver for the same trip for $200 total.

Next was when we went to visit the tombs where King Tut was mummified. We had our iPhones taken away by the men who worked in the tombs that said we couldn't take photos, even though everyone had their phones out snapping away. We had to pay him to get our phones back. They were not worried about preserving the tombs or hieroglyphics. They just wanted us to pay for an extra ticket or give them a tip for allowing you to take photos with your phone.

The worst situation was probably when we were at the airport ready to leave Egypt. The fact that we were ready to leave was an understatement. Clearly, we were ready to get out of there after 10 days of torture. We were so emotionally exhausted at that point and had nothing left in us to argue anymore.

Our taxi had dropped us off at the wrong terminal at about 3:30 a.m., and there was no one around but a guard. He was trying to tell us in very broken English that we were in the wrong place. Then he insisted that we pay him $10 in exchange for calling us a taxi to take us to the other terminal. We declined his service, and as we walked into the terminal to check the flight board, he started yelling and running after us. We couldn't understand why he was so angry and why he did not want us to enter the terminal.

When we realized that the driver had indeed left us at the wrong airport terminal, we ended up jumping in a car that pulled up to the curb. Out jumped a man, and as he took his luggage out of the trunk, we put our luggage in the trunk. We opened the door to find a lovely French couple. The couple was living in Egypt for work, and they were not surprised when we told them our story. They were kind people and refused to accept money to drive us to the other terminal.

Naturally, when the EgyptAir airplane took off to head towards Tunisia, we couldn't help but do a little dance to celebrate. I never have wanted to leave a country so bad in my life. I felt exhausted, abused, worn-down, and defeated. Every place we went to was a fight. Going to Egypt made me grateful for the freedom I have as a woman and the freedom I have to say NO and not be bothered or questioned for saying it.

LESSONS LEARNED

Traveling to a new country has lots of unknowns. Not all countries have the same values as you and may treat you differently. Egypt is not as cool as it appears, so enter with caution. Be aware of your surroundings and listen to your gut when you travel to a new place. Your gut always knows best. And don't forget to love yourself, no matter what country you go to.

CAPÍTULO SIETE: CACHAÇA COM MEL

After the *Plaza de España*, we headed back to the hotel. We were jetlagged and tired from walking around the city, and it was time to take a break. I was really enjoying my time with Anderson, and I could tell that he loved Seville too, so I was pleased.

We walked back hand in hand to the *Plaza de Encarnaciòn*, where the strange wooden structure that they had built in 2010 called *Las Setas,* or "the mushrooms," stood. Our hotel was located directly behind it. As we walked up to the *Setas*, we heard a loud noise and lots of music. It sounded like a band procession from *Semana Santa*, and as we approached, we saw a big float of the Virgin Mary filled with candles and men underneath the float were carrying it.

Seeing the float of the Virgin Mary brought me back to 2006 when I was living in Sao Joao do Oriente, a small town in Minas Gerais, Brazil. I was married to Walter at the time, and we were visiting his family for two weeks. During the time we were there, the *Festa Juninha* was going on. The *Festa Juninha* was an annual festival in the town with lots of traditional foods, dance, and alcohol. This took place every June outside in the main plaza of the small town where they lived. I was super excited to experience it for the first time, because all of our friends from Sao Joao do Oriente back home in Massachusetts were always talking about it and sharing their favorite memories from when they were kids. *Forró* (pronounced fo-ho) was a traditional dance from Minas Gerais, and Walter had even won a *Forró* dance contest there as a child.

Walter and I got dressed and went downtown to the plaza, where we met his brother and his wife. As usual when I went out on the town, everyone stared at me, because I was clearly not from there, and I did not look like everyone else who lived there. Being a tall, 5'9, overweight, blonde woman with a funny Portuguese accent did not help me blend in. I always felt so awkward in big groups, because it was clear that people would whisper and talk about "*a Americana*" (the American girl).

We decided to walk around and watch some of the dance contests happening on the stage. Naturally, we decided to buy some drinks. We arrived at a stand that had a big sign that said, "*Cachaça Com Mel*," but I didn't see any drinks. Instead, the stand had a bunch of plastic-like tubes that looked like straws that were lined up that had a green and yellow substance inside.

"What's this?" I asked.

Walter responded, "Oh, it's *cachaça com mel.*"

I knew *cachaça* was the famous Brazilian tequila that was locally made, and *mel* was honey. I had never seen anything like this before, but I decided to try it. Most Brazilian drinks and treats were delicious, even if the combination wasn't something that I was used to, so we each bought one.

The *cachaça com mel* was in a big, long, plastic tube that was about the length of my body in size. It reminded me of a liquid pixie stick. The vendor cut open the top, and we did a *brinde* (cheers) and sucked down the first gulp. Immediately, a tingly warm, strong taste went running through my body. I LOVED IT. The mixture of honey with the tequila made it go down so smoothly, and I loved the high sensation I felt from the tequila. I felt like I was floating. And so the adventure began.

We walked around and watched the different shows and processions throughout the town and even did some dancing of our own. The plaza was super crowded with hundreds of people, and we said hello to the familiar faces and to Walter's family members who had also come down to the festival.

Walter tried to teach me *forró*, but at that point, I was feeling quite drunk. I tried my best to dance *forró* the American way. As the night went on, we kept going back to get more cachaça com mel, because they were only two Reais, which was about 50 cents in USD.

After a few hours, I started to feel strange. Really, I couldn't feel much at all. I felt almost numb, and I started vomiting. All of a sudden, I found myself alone in town, removed from the party, sitting and crying on someone's doorstep behind the festival. Somehow, I had lost track of Walter, his brother, and his wife, and I didn't know where I was or how I was going to get home.

After sitting by myself for a while and swaying back and forth, Walter appeared out of nowhere. He came across very angry and frustrated.

"Where have you been?" he said. "I have been looking everywhere for you. I was worried about where you had gone and what happened to you."

I don't know what hit me inside, but I got angry, and we started arguing. "I'm totally fine," I said in a slurred speech. "You don't have to baby me. I can take care of myself. I know what I am doing," I replied. As soon as I said those words, I fell over and fainted. Thank God Walter was standing right there, because he stopped me from hitting my head.

I kept going in and out of consciousness, and the next thing I remember was vaguely being picked up off of the stoop by two men and being put into a wheelchair. In my drunken state, I remember feeling like a burden to them as a 250-pound American girl who could not hold her liquor. The two men were pushing me in the wheelchair over the cobblestone road towards the infirmary, which was closed because of the festival. I could feel myself getting nauseous again as the wheels hit the cobblestones.

Eventually I completely passed out and woke up 2 hours later laying in the infirmary with an IV in my arm. Walter and his brother had picked me up and pushed me in the wheelchair to the clinic where they had been watching me over the last couple of hours. They had been able to locate a doctor in town, and he kindly came to open the clinic to help me. The only thing that I remember from the clinic was laying there with an IV in my arm with a light so strong that it was blinding me, so I laid with my eyes closed.

I can't even remember how I got home that morning. I just remember waking up in Walter's parents' bed, wondering how I had arrived there. There were two things that surrounded me: vomit and shame. I was so embarrassed.

Why did Walter put me in his parents' bed? Why was I here by myself? What day was it? What time was it? How long had I been asleep? Why did my head hurt so much? Where did Walter's parents sleep? All of these questions flooded my mind until I heard a knock on the door. Walter came in, and he looked very stern and serious.

"I know. I disappointed you," I said. "I am so embarrassed about what happened last night. How am I going to face your parents?"

Walter just stared at me like one of the towns people who had never seen a tall blonde American before.

"What?" I said, as I stared back.

"Are you ok?" he asked.

"I think so," I replied. "Shame is the biggest thing that I am feeling right now."

"You should be," he said. "You could have been seriously injured. Do you know that the closest hospital is over an hour away from here? What if we couldn't wake you up?"

I was quiet as I felt my eyes well up with tears. "I don't even know how I got so drunk," I said as I sobbed.

Walter replied, "*cachaça com mel.*"

I have no recollection of how many of those tubes that I consumed. Walter said that I had at least 4 big tubes before I disappeared, and who knows what else I had after I separated from him and his brother. He told me that I said that I was going to the bathroom, and I never returned.

I was so disappointed in myself. *How could I have allowed myself to get to a drunken state like this, again?* I could tell that Walter was getting tired of it, and I had to figure something out. Sure, I liked having a good time, but this had gone beyond having a good time.

I will have to learn how to control my alcohol better, I thought to myself. And with that thought, I stood up to go out and face Walter's parents.

Later that year, as my drinking got worse, Walter ended up convincing me to attend an AA meeting. He went with me the first couple times because I was terrified. I didn't end up staying in AA at that time, but the seed had been planted and I knew where I needed to go years later when my life fell apart due to alcohol.

LESSONS LEARNED

If you can't control your drinking, or any substance, it is okay to ask for help. Using other substances to soothe yourself is not a healthy way to deal with problems or uncomfortable emotions. Alcohol is dangerous when it is abused, and *cachaça com mel* is deadly. Have the courage to admit you have a problem and the desire to change it. Love yourself, by putting healthy food and drinks into your body instead of things like cachaça com mel.

CAPÍTULO OCHO: WHY DOESN'T MONEY GROW ON TREES?

After Anderson and I ate lunch, we took a *siesta*! We really needed a nap after barely sleeping on the long overnight flight. *Man, I love the Spanish culture,* I thought. While the Spanish economy was not flourishing and booming, they sure knew how to live life to the fullest.

After our nap, I wanted to show Anderson the city center where all of the shops and pedestrian streets were. It was not a far walk from our hotel, so we showered and went out feeling refreshed again. We passed by store after store. Spain definitely had a certain European fashion look, and I loved it. I loved visiting Zara because it was so much cheaper in Spain than the USA. As we walked into Zara, I couldn't help but notice the display table in front of me filled with different styles of jeans. As I stood there and stared at it, it reminded me of my old closet in my apartment in Boston.

As I gazed at my closet in front of me, I said to myself "Is this for real?! How do I have so many jeans?" I started counting the piles and piles of pants that were in front of me. "Twenty-six, twenty-seven, twenty-eight, twenty— Is that two pairs or one pair there?"

What had my life come to? What had my closet come to? Where did I get all of the money to buy these clothes? I thought to myself. Oh, right, my credit card.

Growing up, my mother had always tried to teach me about money, but I was never really interested in learning (clearly). "Remember to save," she would always tell me. "Make a budget so you don't overspend."

I can remember sitting there as a teenager helping my mother pay the bills so that I could learn how to write checks. But budgets and savings never interested me. I always thought that I had the rest of my life ahead of me to learn how to save and worry about money.

I grew up middle class, but my parents always worked very hard for everything that we had. Thankfully, as I got older, my parents' financial situation significantly improved. When my parents got married at 22 and 25 years old, they decided to wait 8 years to have me, their first child. This was so that they could work hard and become more financially stable.

When I was little, we would rarely go out to eat. We would only go if there was a very special occasion to celebrate. If we did go out to eat, we knew we were not allowed to ask for drinks besides tap water unless it was a very, VERY special occasion.

When it came to buying clothes, we often went to discount stores or bought things that were on sale. That, mixed with me being overweight and always a bigger size for my age, made it almost impossible to find clothes that fit me right that I felt good in that were also within budget. And so all of my life, my mindset around money has been scarcity or lacking and always hoping that I have enough. Today, I have worked hard through mindset activities, EFT therapy, and affirmations to change the way that I view money.

So again, how did I end up with 30 pairs of jeans in my closet? My credit card.

As I opened my credit card statement, I cringed at the amount due I saw on the bill. $22,683.72. How could that number be right? I opened up the statement and looked at the purchases over the last month:

*Zara - $103 Why couldn't I buy those clothes at Zara in Spain and save half of the bill!
*Forever 21 - $90.25 Those dresses I got were so cute!
*Hard Rock Café - $60.87 That dinner with Patty was bomb!
*TJ Maxx - $120 Those clothes for work will come in handy.
*Marshalls - $208 These clothes will too.
*John's Liquor Store - $64.87 SUCH a fun party on Friday… Can't wait to do it again!
*TGI Fridays - $47.62 That was a great birthday dinner we had there for Charlie.
*Clark's Bar - $42 They play the best music there.
*Dominos - $22 They have my favorite pizza there! I can taste it now!
*The Cheesecake Factory - $55.99 I love their original cheesecake!
*Jillian's Bar and Bowling - $35.54 Such a fun double date with Mik and Patty
*Joe's Liquor - $78.23 Ah, yes, the party on Saturday. Must plan another one this weekend!

That reminds me, Patty owes me $20 for our dinner at The Hard Rock Cafe, I thought to myself. As if $20 was going to make a dent in my $22,000 bill! Where had all of my money gone? Well, let's see, according to April's Chase Credit Card statement, it went to bars, fast food, alcohol, and clothes.

How did I get this out of control with my spending? My mother had taught me to save and budget, hadn't she?

The sad truth was that this was only one credit card statement. I still had Discover, $10,652.54; Capital One, $9,853.27; and Bank of America, $15,832.44. What was I going to do? How was I going to get out of this debt?

It was the spring of 2008, and I had just separated from my husband, Walter, a couple of months before. He too, had credit cards with exorbitant amounts on them. Walter was working 80 hours a week making $13 an hour, and I rarely saw him. I was working at a cleaning company as an interpreter and a saleswoman, making $32,000 a year. And together, we had accumulated all of this debt.

Walter and I had decided to buy a condo in Worcester, Massachusetts right before the 2008 market crashed. As soon as we bought the home with $0 down, the value of the property dropped, and we soon owed more money to the bank than the home was worth. With two mortgages, a condo fee, and all of the credit card debt we owed, he decided to take his half of the debt and file for bankruptcy.

At first, I was outraged, because we were going to lose our condo, and I thought that if he filed for bankruptcy, it would affect my credit as his wife. But that is what he wanted to do, and the bankruptcy ended up only affecting him. When we separated, I continued to live in the condo until the bank kicked me out, and he took off and moved to Florida. Thankfully, Walter filing for bankruptcy actually wiped out the majority of my debt since a lot of the credit cards were in his name and I was just a second user.

When I opened my business in 2018, the first thing I was told was, get a good accountant. I opened my business, Freelance N' Freedom, with no debt and a clean slate. While I am not the best at sticking to my budget at times, I have learned the value in being organized, having a budget, and keeping track of my finances, especially when it comes to business.

LESSONS LEARNED

Learning how to budget your money can save you a lot of stress in the long run. Make a plan, and only use credit cards for emergencies or items that you pay off monthly. Don't spend money carelessly and dig yourself into a hole like I did. Having limits with money is another form of self-care. And don't forget to love yourself by saying no to things that you cannot afford.

CAPÍTULO NUEVE: WEEKEND GETAWAYS

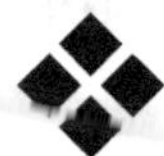

As we walked out of Zara, an old Ford Taurus came flying past us and almost hit an older lady on the corner that was standing next to us. The drivers in Europe like to speed, which can be dangerous when the streets are small and narrow. When the car passed by, it brought me back to my first car.

In my junior year of high school, once I turned 16 and had enough practice driving, my parents handed me down my dad's old green Ford Taurus so I could drive the 30 minutes to school each day. Since I went to a private school outside of our town, I did not have the possibility of taking the school bus.

All of my life, I have been attracted to adventure. I easily get bored doing the same thing over and over, and so I welcome change. I am a Sagittarius, can you tell? When I was a sophomore in high school, I started dating my friend's brother, Earl. Earl was my first boyfriend, and he was two years older than me. He was also the one who introduced me to alcohol and taught me how to party.

Earl decided to go to college in Albany, New York, which was about 2 and a half hours away from where I lived. I was so sad when he chose a college outside of Massachusetts, but we decided to stay together to try to make our relationship work.

Often, my best friend, Patty, and I would go on weekend trips and drive up to Albany to visit Earl. He was in a fraternity, and his fraternity brothers were really fun. Many of them happened to be from Boston. This meant visiting them felt like home and made us comfortable since we all had the same accent and grew up in the same area.

The frat brothers always had fun themed parties, and it was an adventure to make the trek up there in my old green Ford Taurus. Patty and I would take turns driving. It was a straight shot up the Mass Pike on 90 West for two hours. We would tell funny stories to each other, talk about boys in our high school class, and listen to loud, fun 90s music to make the drive go by faster.

My parents would only let me go up and visit Earl once a month at the most, which I did not like. Earl and I went from living 15 minutes away from each other and seeing each other almost every day to living two and a half hours away from each other and seeing each other once a month. That was really difficult, and I wanted to see him more because I missed him so much. Patty enjoyed going up to the fraternity parties just as much as I did, so we decided to come up with a plan.

On Friday night, Patty would ask her parents if she could sleep at my house for the night, and I would ask my parents if I could sleep at Patty's house for the night. This was something that happened regularly anyway, so it was not out of the ordinary. Her parents knew my parents and vice versa. They trusted each other, and so they both usually said yes. We packed a bag, and Patty would leave her car at one of the Massachusetts Turnpike rest stops where it wouldn't get towed, and off we went to Albany.

We went on this adventure many times. We would do it at least once a month, especially when there was a big celebration or party at the fraternity house. If we went on a Friday, oftentimes I would have to work the next day at the Tax Company (my fun high school job) on Saturday. We would leave after school on Friday and get to Albany around 5 or 6 in the afternoon. We would stay until 4 or 5 in the morning and then head home so I could make it to work on time at 8 a.m.

I would show up to work exhausted and often half drunk, but the adventure was so much fun every time. There was something about doing it secretly and getting away with it that also made it fun. Our parents never found out about our adventure trips (until now), and thankfully nothing bad ever happened to us.

LESSONS LEARNED

While I do not encourage you to lie to your parents, I do encourage you to live life to the fullest. You never know when your last adventure will be. Value your close friends, be adventurous, be careful, have fun, and love yourself.

CAPÍTULO DIEZ:
JESUS IS BORN

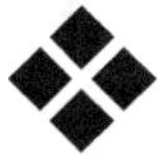

I was super excited to show Anderson the Cathedral of Sevilla. This cathedral is the third largest in the world. It has ruins from Christopher Columbus, and has a ramp that you can hike up 35 floors to the top that looks out over the whole city. Even though we had bought our tickets in advance, there was still a line to get in. The cathedral is made of beautiful Moorish architecture and used to be a mosque back when the Moroccans ruled over southern Spain.

Ding. Dong. Ding. Dong. As we waited in line, the Giralda tower bells started to go off. Waiting in line and hearing the church bells brought me back to my trip to Israel with my friend Mik. It was Christmas Eve in 2016, and we decided to go to Bethlehem in the West Bank to the Church of the Nativity, which was built around the place where they believe that Jesus was born. The Church of the Nativity is a popular place with many tourists from all over the world, so we went with a tour company to cross over the border into Palestine.

Our group was led by an Arab Christian named Peter. After visiting the Shepherds' Fields and another chapel, we headed to the Church of the Nativity, where we found an extremely long line. I mean, it was Christmas Eve, so what else could we expect?

The line circled around inside the church like a snake and went all the way outside, well into Nativity Square. The square was packed with   hundreds of people hanging out and singing Christmas songs around a big Christmas tree. Peter told us that the wait would likely be about 3 hours and asked us if we wanted to stay. We came all this way to Israel, flew 14 hours on a plane, and it was Christmas, so of course we wanted to see where Jesus was born! We decided to suck it up and wait in the line.

Our tour group was rather small with about 10 people. It consisted of a couple from Egypt, a couple from Germany, a family from Australia, and the three of us from the USA. I looked around, and there were much larger tour groups surrounding us in line. We saw a tour group from China, a group of Brits, and the largest group around us was from India.

Before we knew it, the group behind us that was from India became a huge problem. I have yet to travel to India, but after reading other books and hearing other stories, I realized what was about to happen was a big cultural wake up call. They had no personal space boundaries at all, which, you can imagine, became very annoying while waiting in line. Our group of 10 was in front of their group of about 150 people, and they were eager to push the line forward.

The people in the front of their line would get very close to our group in line and surround us in a circle. They would get so close that they would almost be on top of whomever from our group was at the back of the line and not allow room for any personal space. After about 30 minutes, the back of the Indian group started pushing our group. We had to yell at them to stop, and soon enough, Peter went and found their tour guide and addressed the issue with them.

But it didn't really help. This cycle of actions continued for about two hours. Every time the line would move forward, a big wave from the back would start pushing and the group of Indians would run into us. It was like a big tidal wave.

Calm down, we are all going to see where Jesus was born, I thought.

It got very frustrating, and no matter how much we yelled at them, they would not back up.

"Stop!" we yelled. "Back up and give us room!" we insisted.

But they didn't listen, and it seemed as if they almost started to panic. At one point, I could feel them breathing down my neck.

Our tour guide, Peter, had to get involved numerous times. He went at least 5 times to speak to their tour guide. It was so uncomfortable, and it made me start to think about India and what it must be like to live there. Being from a country with millions and millions of people where you have to fight for everything must be such a different and difficult way to live.

I tried to be compassionate to this group of people, until out of nowhere, my thoughts were interrupted by a big push from the back of the line as my body went flying forward. *That's it! I have had it,* I thought.

We were approaching the area where you enter to see where Jesus was born. There was a small set of stairs that led down into a cave-like hole that was very narrow that you had to enter single-file.

How are we all going to fit in here single file with everyone pushing? I thought.

The pushing got so bad that someone almost fell down the stairs. All of a sudden, Peter lifted his arms in the air like a policeman and yelled, "STOP!"

The church went silent, and you could hear his voice echo. Everyone stopped moving.

After a few choice words from Peter, we finally were able to get through. He made sure that everyone in our group entered the little door before the Indian group started to file in behind us.

Inside was very warm and crowded, but also very peaceful. How cool it was to think that I was somewhere in the vicinity of where Jesus was believed to have been born! Although the guard rushed us through because of the long line, it was a mystical moment that I will never forget.

Lessons Learned: Traveling to foreign countries requires patience and an open mind. If you have traveled to destinations with lots of tourists, you have likely experienced this in one way or another. Be patient with other cultures who have different rules about personal space and waiting in lines. And love yourself by not putting yourself in harm's way when you travel.

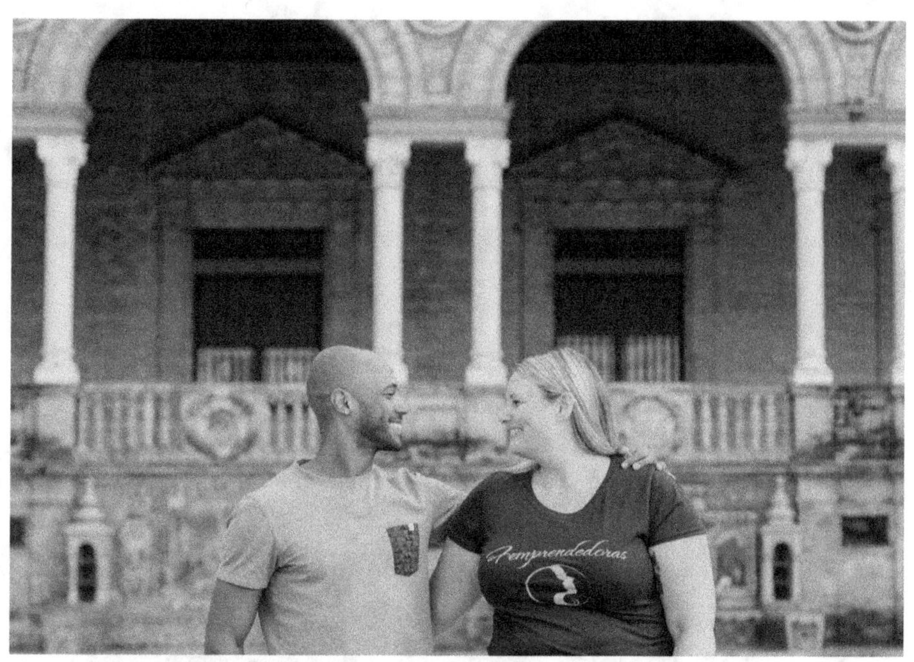

Anderson and I on our trip to Seville visiting the Plaza de España. Photo was taken by Arancha Morera.

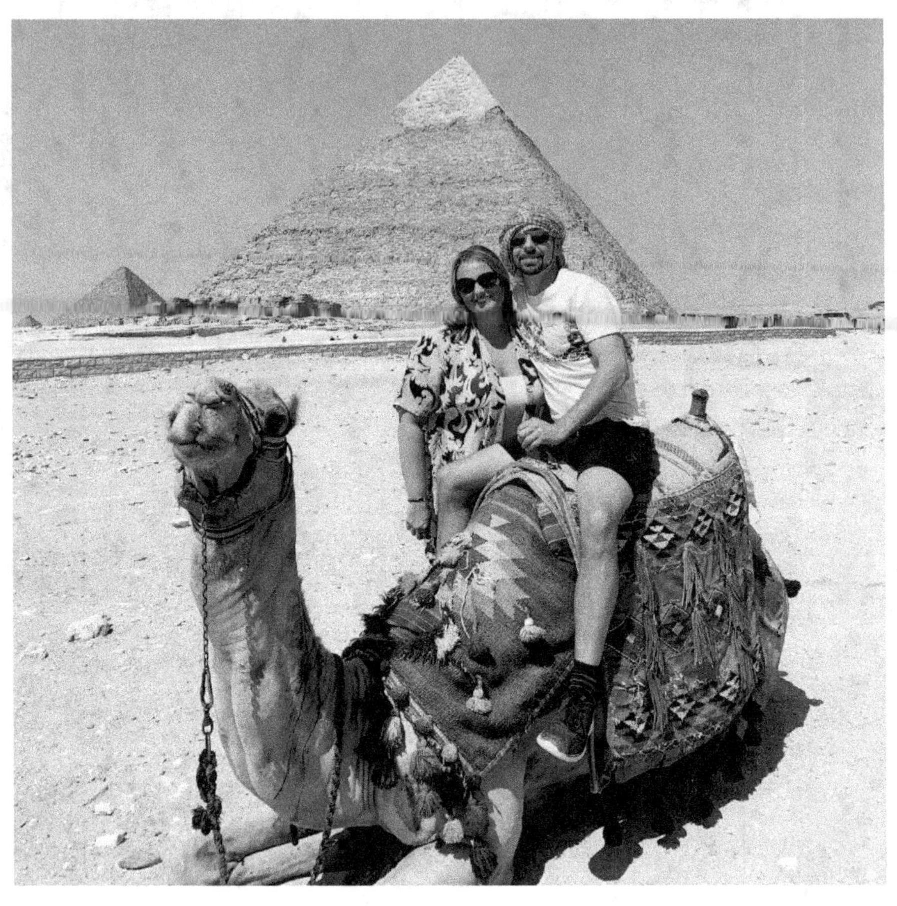

Mik and I on our trip to Egypt taking photos with the camel.

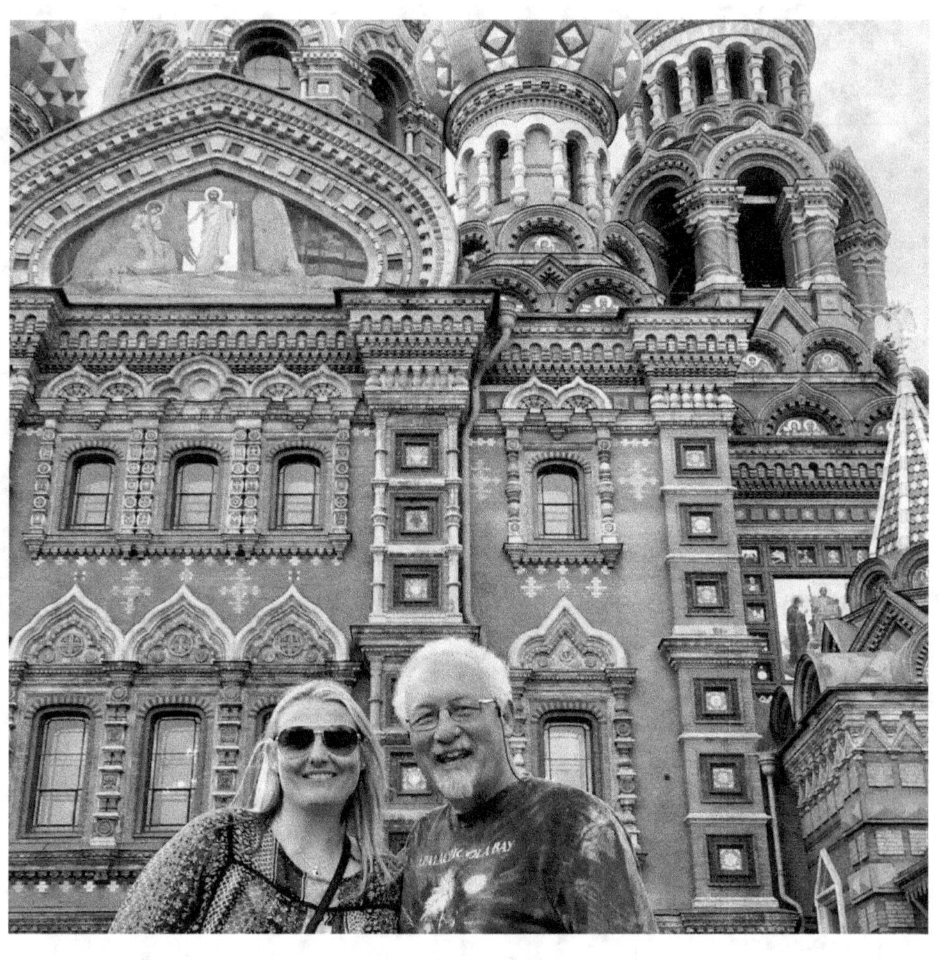

Dad and I on our trip to Scandinavia and Russia after I left Ahmed.

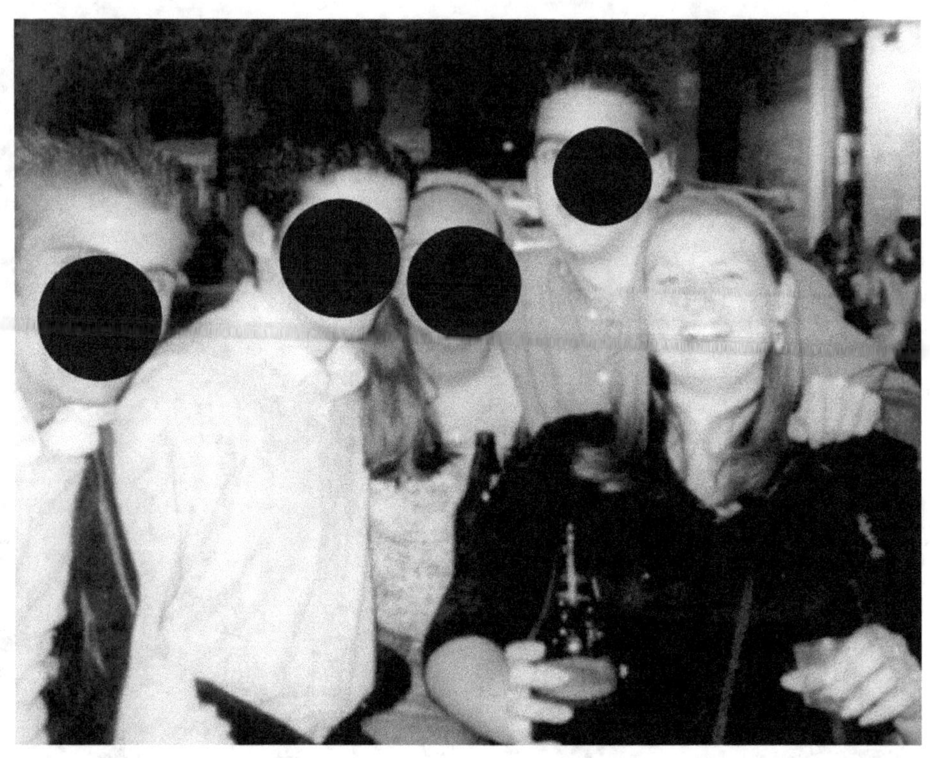

Me partying double-fisted with a group of friends in Seville, Spain when I studied abroad.

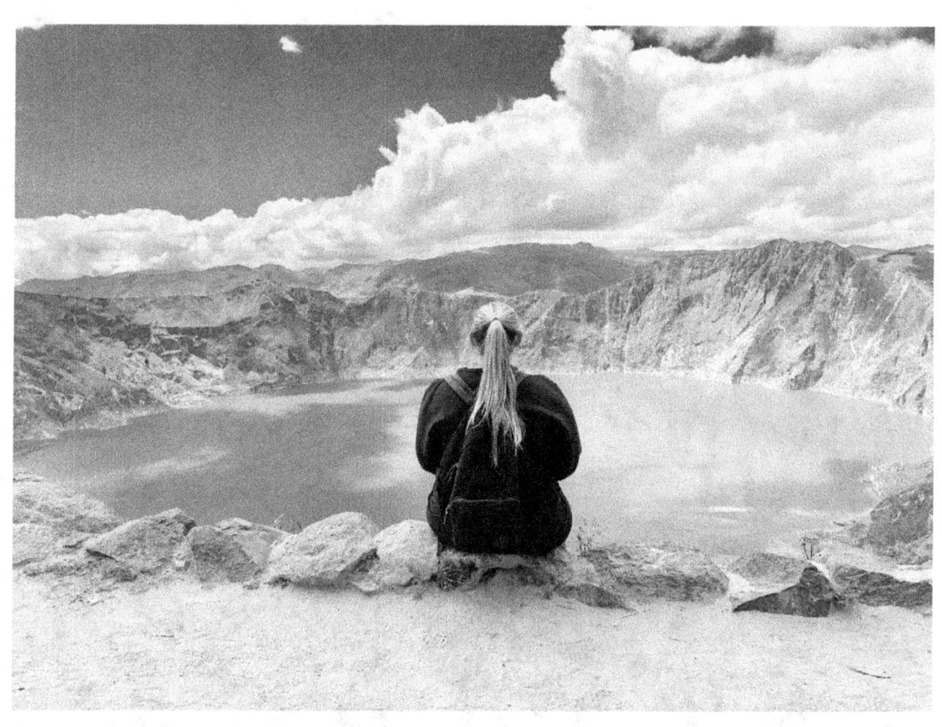

On a solo trip to Ecuador in my first year of traveling the world as an entrepreneur.

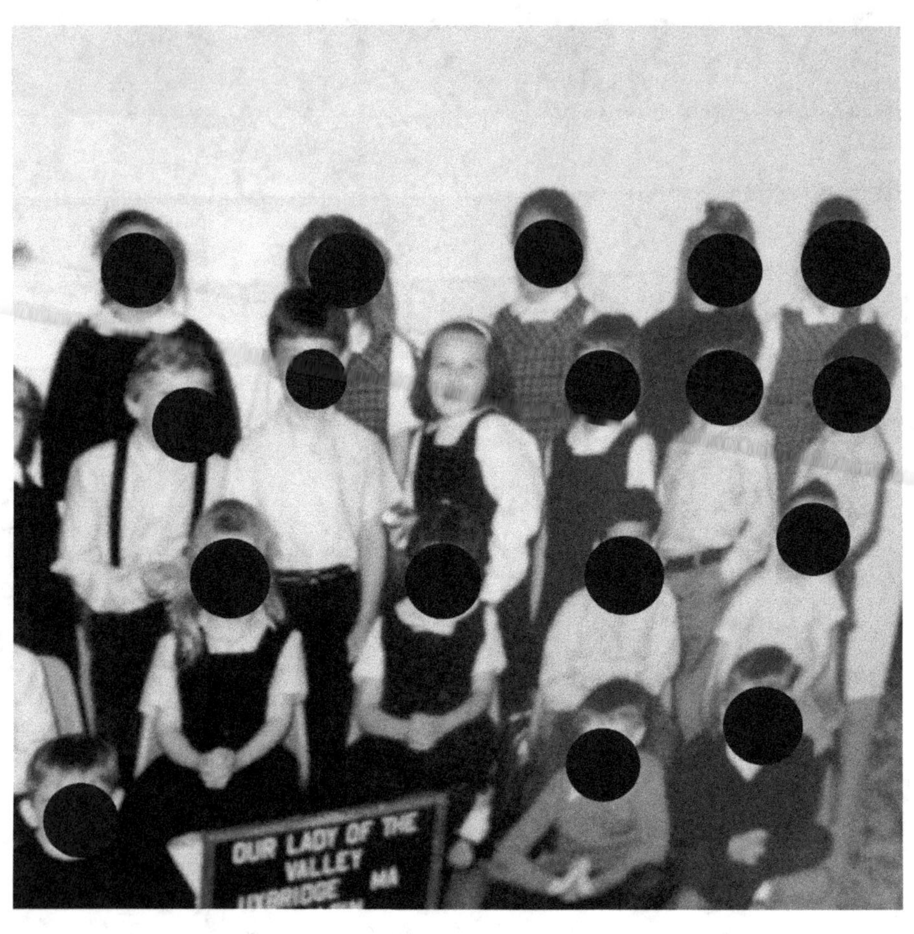

My Kindergarten class photo with Matty Jones (my first love)
and Scott Powers (my first kiss).

CAPÍTULO ONCE: DRINKING AND SLIDING

As we came out of the Cathedral, rain started to come down, and soon it was pouring heavily. It was unusual for it to rain in Seville, so I was surprised and a little disappointed.

Of course it is raining! I thought. It is sunny 300 days a year here and when we decide to come, it rains.

We pulled out the umbrella and ducked under a storefront across from the Cathedral.

As we stood under the awning of the store and the rain poured down relentlessly, the sound of the rain hitting the ground brought me back to my drinking days. Back then, nothing stopped me from going out to get alcohol. No rain or snowstorm could keep me from getting my fix. Oh, what a horrible way to live that was! A sense of gratitude came over me for realizing that I no longer had to leave my home to get what I was addicted to everyday and, especially, in rain or snowstorms.

The rain pouring down on the glass storefront made me remember a specific evening when I was living just outside of Boston with my boyfriend, Marc. As mentioned earlier, we had a crazy connection, and I swore that he was the love of my life, but I am now convinced that our connection revolved around our love for alcohol and our addictive personalities.

One particular summer evening, we had gone out to meet some of his friends at a bar downtown, about a mile from our house. Marc was his usual funny self, until he started drinking whiskey. Once he had a few shots of whiskey in him, he turned into a mean boyfriend. It was the whiskey that completely changed his personality and turned him into a complete psycho.

Why am I with him again? I thought. Oh, right, because I love him.

My relationship with Marc began shortly after my breakup with Walter… a month later to be exact. I had met Marc out at a Brazilian *forró* bar on a Sunday night, where I had gotten completely wasted, because I wanted to escape the reality that my first marriage had ended. I headed out for a night with the girls, and Marc came up to me as I was waiting for a shot at the bar. We ended up hanging out all night, until the next day, when I was scheduled to report to work at the law office at 10 a.m.

The next morning when I went to leave for work, I realized that I had gone to the bar with my girlfriend, Lu, and had forgotten my keys at her house. That meant that I couldn't drive my car. Marc and his friend kindly agreed to drive me all around Massachusetts: first home, (which was 45 minutes away) so I could change my clothes and not go to work looking like I had just left the club, and then to my friend's house where I had left my keys the night before (another 45 minutes), and then to work (another 1.5 hours in traffic). Needless to say, I didn't arrive at work until about 11:30, but it wasn't a busy day, and I told the lawyer that I worked for that I had been locked out of my car (which was kind of true).

Marc and my relationship continued to grow and flourish, because we both had the same love: alcohol. Basically our whole relationship revolved around it, especially on the weekends. We would start drinking Friday right after work and not stop until late Sunday night or early Monday morning. This pattern continued for months, and months turned into years.

And that rainy Friday night was no different. Marc had started with the whiskey before he had even left work, and so although the night was young, he started to call me names. He was, yet again, mad over nothing. I was tired of him treating me poorly and did not want to cause a scene, so I suggested that we go home. Sometimes changing the location would cause Marc to forget that he was "angry" at me, and he would go back to being a nice guy again. Plus, it was embarrassing in front of our friends for him to sit there and say bad things about me that weren't true, just because he had some whiskey.

I was pretty drunk, and Marc insisted he was fine to drive. I handed him the keys to my '98 bright blue Chevy Cavalier that was a gift given to me by my grandmother before she had to go into a nursing home. As we walked out to the car, the rain started to come down hard, and we started to run. Marc started the engine and pulled out of the parking lot in a rush.

"Slow down!" I yelled at him.

As I looked over at Marc, his face looked like a guy that had gone mad. He was holding the steering wheel with two hands, and his eyes were popping out of his head like a crazy man. He had this strange grin on his face as he was speeding down the road.

The rain continued pouring down, lightning flashed, and I could not see anything out of the front windshield.

If I can't see anything, how can he? I thought.

Marc didn't even have a driver's license due to his legal status, and he was driving like a bat out of hell.

As I turned to look back at the street, I realized that Marc was driving on the wrong side of the road! My heart jumped in my throat, and I started to yell! "Maaaarc! What are you doing?"

I looked at him again, and he still had that crazy look in his eyes as he gripped the steering wheel. I tried yelling again, but it seemed as if something had control over him.

Suddenly, through the big drops of rain, there appeared a bright light shining towards us. I thought to myself, *this could be it.*

I yelled at Marc and said, "What are you doing?! You're on the wrong side of the road!"

Finally, he snapped out of it and swerved to go back on the right side of the road. As we slid across the pavement and hydroplaned, a four-wheeler truck stormed by us and honked his horn. Marc pulled over and stopped the car. We were both breathing heavily and looked at each other.

I said, "Marc, you almost just killed us."

He remained silent and just stared straight ahead at the pouring rain coming down on the windshield.

If a near death experience doesn't sober you up, I don't know what will. I demanded that he get out and let me drive the half a mile we had to get home. I drove us home in silence and pulled into the driveway. It was still pouring rain, and I ran inside the house as fast as I could. Marc couldn't even look me in the face, and I crawled into bed and passed out in my wet clothes.

LESSONS LEARNED

Don't drink and drive. Drinking and driving takes many innocent lives every year and causes devastation to families and individuals who survive accidents. It is not worth the risk and putting yourself and others in danger. You are worth love, patience, and respect. Love yourself, and don't let anyone mistreat you, bully you, or put you down, no matter who they are.

CAPÍTULO DOCE: LUCKY LINZ

The next day, Anderson and I decided to go on a day trip. We got on the Renfe train to head to Ronda for the day to visit my old roommate, Antonio, who had recently had a baby. I lived with Antonio when I was teaching English before I met Ahmed. I love Europe for its amazing public transportation system. It is cheap and effective, and you can travel from country to country efficiently and inexpensively.

As the train started to move and I stared out the window, it reminded me of my backpacking trip through Europe with my friend, Mik. It was 2003, and my parents had given me a Eurail train pass for Christmas before I left to study abroad in Seville. At the end of my semester of school in May, I met Mik in Madrid to take the train to various countries for 2 weeks. We didn't even have a plan really, just a map and a guidebook.

At 20 years old, I couldn't believe our parents were letting us do this on our own, but I was filled with excitement and wonder! This was also the trip that really sparked the travel bug in me, since we visited 7 countries in 20 days.

I met Mik in Madrid after taking the overnight bus from Seville. I always hated that bus. It was so uncomfortable, especially when it was crowded, because there was no leg room to stretch out. This was nothing new as my 5'9 height was not in my favor when it came to public transportation. 7 hours on a bus with a few stops is a nightmare, especially for light sleepers like me, but it was all I could afford at the time.

I caught a taxi from the bus station that took me to our hostel. Even though it was only 7:30 a.m., I had this funny feeling that someone was watching me. When I looked up at the window, there was Mik filming me on his video camera.

Let the fun begin, I thought.

Mik and I had known each other for 5 years at that point. (Today, we have been friends for over 23 years). He was always up to playing games, cracking jokes, and making fun out of whatever miserable situation we were in. And today was no different.

After a 7-hour overnight bus ride cramped with an elderly woman next to me and probably an hour of sleep, Mik had made sure he was up at 7:30 a.m. to greet me and welcome my beautiful face with filming on his camera. I am sure that I looked horrible, but I looked up at him, smiled, and waved.

And so the trip commenced. After a couple of days in Madrid, our first stop was France. We headed up to Paris on the overnight train from Madrid for a few days. Little did we know that the hostel we had booked did not have a shower, just a sink in the room. I guess it is true what they say: French people don't like to shower! Sponge bath it is! We managed and made the best we could of it.

After a few days in Paris, we headed to Amsterdam. We did not stay there for long, since we were offered cocaine getting off of the overnight train at 7 a.m. and all of the cafés around us allowed for weed smoking, which we were not into. We knew Amsterdam was known for being liberal when it came to drugs, but it was an uncomfortable place to be. We had had enough when we bought sandwiches, and they started charging us 2 euros for a small package of ketchup. We did, however, enjoy the Anne Frank Huis museum there.

From Amsterdam, we headed to Krakow, Poland, then Prague, Czech Republic, until we got to Switzerland. From Switzerland, we headed to Germany, and our last stop would be Italy to visit Mik's family.

On our way to Germany, we had to make a stop in Linz, Austria. In Linz, we would get off and catch a connecting train that would bring us into Germany. At this point, we were about halfway through the trip, and we had just spent a few days in Switzerland. We were both exhausted and at the point in our trip where we were both a bit homesick and tired of sleeping on trains. Traveling on a train for two weeks with only a backpack, sometimes in a bed, while other times in a seat, was very daunting on your body, even at age 20. We still look back at that trip today and realize we could never backpack that way now in our thirties.

On this leg of the trip specifically, we were not able to reserve a room for us to sleep in, and our train was arriving in Linz at 2 a.m.

We decided that we would take turns sleeping so that we would not miss our stop. I remember the train had blue seats and was freezing cold. I hate when they blast the air, especially at night. We had a set of four seats to ourselves that were so hard and uncomfortable, and we didn't have any blankets. It is difficult for me to fall asleep in any place that is cold or uncomfortable. I would much rather be in a warm environment.

I should have set the boundary with Mik that he would sleep for a certain amount of time and then we would switch. As I thought about this, Mik crawled onto the floor under the four seats and said he was going to take a little nap until we got to Linz. And just like that, he was out like a light.

Ugh, I thought. *I am so exhausted and need to get some sleep too.* I could feel myself getting angry as I looked at Mik asleep on the floor rolled up in a ball. Mik and I have always been good friends; however, we also have been known to get on each other's nerves at times, especially when traveling.

I found myself dozing on and off in the chair and trying my hardest to keep my eyes open. I tried yelling at Mik to wake up so that I could have a little nap, but he did not move. He was out cold. We did not have iPhones back then to set an alarm either.

All of a sudden, I felt the train jolt. The train came to a halting stop, and I opened my eyes. I looked on the floor, and Mik was still there sleeping, snug as a bug. I was so annoyed that he wouldn't take his turn and let me get some sleep. He had been sleeping the whole time.

Speaking of time… What time is it?

I stood up and looked out the window to try to see the name of the stop. I could not see the name anywhere. All of the signs were in German. I was able to wake up Mik, and he was all out of sorts and seemed very confused.

"Where are we? Are we in Linz? What time is it?" he asked.

I got mad immediately that he had taken the liberty to sleep for as long as he wanted and had not given me the chance to take a nap. I felt the frustration inside me rise up through my body, but I was too tired to say anything. Just as I was going to start scolding him, the train started to move. We ran through to the next train car and pressed ourselves up against the window. As the train started moving, we saw the sign out of the window: LINZ.

"No, this can't be happening! We are missing our stop! No! Stop!" we started to yell, but it was too late.

It reminded me of a scene from a movie, except it was happening to us in real life. As we stood there with our bags, we saw all of the signs that said LINZ on them passing us by.

"Ugh, this is so frustrating!" I said to Mik.

"Yeah, why didn't you wake me up?" he said.

I could feel my face turning red with rage. My entire body got hot, but honestly at that point I had no energy in me to argue with him because it was 2 a.m., and I was exhausted. The only thing I could afford was a strong, dirty stare.

I decided to let it go, and I stood up to find one of the crew members to ask what the next stop was and how far away we were from it. As I walked through the train cars looking for a member of the staff, pretty much everyone I walked by was fast asleep.

Lucky bastards, I thought to myself.

When I finally found one of the train crew, I asked, "Excuse me, sir… What is the next stop, and how far is it?"

The man responded, "The next stop is Horn, Austria, and it is two and a half hours from here, dear."

"2 and a half hours!" I exclaimed. "No way! With all due respect, sir, do you mean to tell me that there is not one stop from Linz to Horn? We missed our stop in Linz and need to get off to turn around."

"I am sorry, dear. There is no other stop on this route until Horn."

If it was not 2:30 in the morning, I would have probably screamed. I could not believe what I was hearing.

What are we going to do? I thought.

I headed back to our car to tell Mik the great news. He was going to be thrilled.

LESSONS LEARNED

When you are traveling, make sure you plan ahead so you know where you are going. It is okay to set boundaries with those you travel with. Take turns, take care of yourself, get enough sleep, and love yourself.

CHAPTER TRECE: TWENTY-FOUR/SEVEN

Anderson and I arrived in Ronda after a few hours on the train. We had so much fun there. It was so good to see Antonio, his wife, and new daughter after so many years. I hadn't been to Ronda since my school trip in college when I studied abroad. The huge gorge in the center of the city was such a magnificent and breathtaking site to see. We spent the day with Antonio and his wife as our guide, walking through the little narrow streets and alleys of Ronda. They took us to their favorite restaurant and showed us the church where they got married. They brought us to the famous ham market where the slices melt in your mouth like butter.

Anderson and I headed back to Seville the same evening on the train. As we boarded and sat in our seats, I looked over at the gentleman sitting next to us, who was typing on his laptop.

In 2021, the society we live in is full of technology, smart phones, laptops, tablets, PlayStation, iWatches, and whatever electronic device that is hot on the market. In 2018, I left my job at Harvard University for various reasons. The main one was so that I could travel and run my business from wherever I wanted that had a Wi-Fi signal.

How lucky am I?! I thought to myself. I have the ability to work from the beach, a café, a coworking space with cool friends, or whatever country I am in! This is so cool.

Or so I thought. As time went on and I began working full-time as a virtual assistant, I realized that being able to work from anywhere was not as fun as I thought. My idea of working virtually from the photos that I had seen on Instagram was far from the truth. After I went from having three clients part-time to working for myself full-time, I suddenly found myself with eight clients. And eight clients were way too many. I was working constantly, 24/7, and was receiving emails and texts at all hours of the day and night.

My first year as an entrepreneur, I set the goal to travel to a new country every month. Living in Miami affords you the proximity to South and Central America, the Caribbean Islands, and cheap flights. So, I started my year going to Jamaica, then Panama, then Guatemala, and Costa Rica. Then in April, I headed back to Spain to Barcelona and Ibiza with my sister and did a side trip to the small country of Andorra. This was followed by a trip to Egypt and Tunisia with Mik in May. June was Ecuador, and in July I went to Northern Ireland, the Isle of Man, and Scotland. In August and September, I took a break, and in October and November I went back to Spain again. I finished the year in December with the Spain and Israel trips with Anderson.

Traveling to new countries while I was working added a layer of difficulty to the work with clients in different time zones and wanting to see the new cities I was in. Travelling to different countries really tested my boundaries. I would try to set up a routine for myself. However, I would often find myself texting or responding to emails while I was in the street of whatever country I was in, and I would get stressed and frustrated with limited internet service.

Whether I was walking through the streets of Ecuador, on one of the San Blas Islands of Panama, or riding through the Highlands of Scotland, I would get texts and emails at all hours of the day and night. The expectation was always that I would have to answer as quickly as possible.

What was the point of traveling to all of these new places if I couldn't enjoy them? How did I get to this point and why is this happening? I thought.

Working for myself was not turning out to be as fun as Instagram had made it seem. One night as I was lying in bed and texting a client back at 11 p.m., I thought, *What am I doing?!* It suddenly clicked as I was responding that this was why my clients expected that I responded to them immediately and at all hours of the day and night.

Hello, Christine, you are responding at 11 p.m. You are showing clients how you want to be treated.

From that moment, I decided that I could not continue working and traveling this way anymore.

I decided to make a plan. I would email my clients and tell them that I was not going to be answering them after 5 PM or on the weekends, and I said that if they needed anything urgent from me, to ask before then. And then I just stopped responding at strange times. In the beginning of being a business owner, the way I saw it was that I always had work to do, so if I responded immediately, that would be one less thing that I had on my list to do. But the truth is, as an entrepreneur, you always have work to do, so it doesn't matter if you respond at 11 p.m. or wait until the morning to get back to them, because 9 out of 10 times, it is not urgent.

I also made the decision that 8 clients was really too many to balance at once for a one-woman company, unless I decided to outsource or hire help, which I did not want to do at the time. I went from 8 clients to 6, and after a couple of more months, I let go of two more, and went from 6 to 4. Four clients seemed to be a good number that I could balance and make enough income from, while allowing me to also have time for self-care and not answering emails and texts at all hours of the day.

I also committed to using a color-coordinated Google calendar and plan out each day on it, including time for working out, meditation, journaling and taking breaks for lunch. This has helped me tremendously and has allowed me to set healthy boundaries so that I am not always working. I went through a time at the beginning of 2021 that I was no longer working on Fridays. I let my clients know of my schedule change, and if I ended up doing any work, it is work for myself, and not meetings, calls, or clients.

LESSONS LEARNED

Nothing is as good as it seems. If working and traveling were as easy as it looks on Instagram, everyone would do it. If you work for yourself, it is important to set boundaries around your working hours, your schedule, working on the weekends, and when you respond to texts and emails, especially when you are just starting out. Communicate the boundaries clearly to those who you work with. As a business owner, there is always going to be work to do. Love yourself by setting reasonable routines and boundaries so that you can have a great work/life balance.

CAPÍTULO CATORCE: VITAL MARKETING

Our vacation was going by so fast! The next day, we decided to do some souvenir shopping and explore the center of the city. We loved walking, and so Anderson and I set out towards Calle Sierpes, which was the main street in the shopping district. I inhaled the Seville air and fell in love all over again as the sweet smell of azahar filled my nostrils. As we walked downtown, we turned the corner near the University of Sevilla and ran into a huge crowd of people. Many of them were holding flags and yelling words in Spanish.

What is going on? I thought.

Of course, it was a manifestation, or *huelga*, as they liked to call it in Spain. From an outsider, one would think that this was strange or dangerous with more than 1000 people in the street yelling with signs. But actually this was your typical Spanish afternoon, and the protesting was peaceful and frequent.

Spain is very big on demonstrating and fighting for their rights, especially the students. I remembered when I studied at the University of Sevilla, once or twice a month there were *huelgas*, which meant, no class. I remember the excitement that I felt every time I would arrive at the university, only to find that class was cancelled due to a protest. I already did not have class on Fridays, so I often would only have to go to class three days a week. A lot of times, I think the students just demonstrated to get out of going to class and that the demonstration wasn't really something they believed in. They would sit in the middle of Calle San Fernando and chant and yell and block the cars going by.

I remember there being lots of *huelgas* about the Spanish president. There was the the trash strike, teachers' pay, students' rights, women's equal pay, the war on Iraq, and so the list went on.

All of the chanting and yelling that I heard brought me back to my first job after I graduated college. It was 2005, and I had been hired to work as an account manager for Maxwell Solutions (named after John Maxwell, the famous writer on leadership) in Braintree, Massachusetts.

The owner of the company was Sun Chang, a 25-year-old, 6'2", Korean man who was full of energy and jokes. Sun was an amazing motivator and salesmen and someone who cheered me on and believed in me, even when I did not believe in myself.

Maxwell Solutions was a pyramid scheme sales business. It partnered with and sold products for companies like Verizon, Quill Office Supply, the local electric company, and others. You would enter the business as an account manager doing door-to-door sales. Then you would be promoted to a lead account manager and still do door-to-door sales. Then become an assistant manager to learn the behind the scenes of running a business, and then a manager or owner of your own company.

The last part was really what intrigued me. This was my first attempt at being an entrepreneur. In about a year, I could build a team and a business and be the owner of my own company at age 23! All I had to do was become a great saleswoman and build a team of people who wanted to follow me and support me to open up my own office. My goal was to open Vital Marketing, because at the time, I was engaged to be married to Walter, and *Vital* would become my new last name.

I took my job very seriously. Every morning, I arrived between 6:45 and 7 a.m., which meant that I had to leave my house at 5:45 a.m. I would dress in some kind of a suit, or jacket and pants, and arrive to set up and get ready for the day. I treated the office there as if it were mine, because I really wanted to learn the behind the scenes of running a business.

Every morning, we would gather for the kickoff meeting at 7:20 a.m., and Sun would start to blast music and yell to get us hyped up for the day, much like the huelga in Spain. He would chant, give some kind of inspirational speech on how to be an amazing leader (think *Wolf of Wall Street*), and announce the top salespeople from the day before to our entire office.

Believe it or not, I often was number 1 in the country out of thousands of sales reps! Yes, me, Christine Seibold, would go out each day and sell my ass off so that I could be seen on the list as number one in the country the next morning.

Our office would frequently attend various sales conferences. People would recognize my name on my nametag and know it from being announced at the top of the sales list in their offices all over the country. At age 22, this was really all that I cared about: recognition and making money (and partying, of course). I even received a leadership award my first year in the company in front of thousands of people, and let me tell you, it felt amazing.

Even though my job was 100% commission, I loved it, and I loved the people I worked with. Most of them were in their early 20s and had just graduated college. I made great relationships there, and it was really fun.

The best part was that we hung out outside of work, too. There was always a sales conference in New England or Philadelphia that we attended every couple of months, and every

Thursday night was team night, which meant beer, wings, and pizza on the boss. Whatever the event was, there was lots of drinking included, which, of course, I loved. The weekends were spent at Sun's house playing beer pong and other drinking games and watching movies, which totally complimented my drinking lifestyle at the time.

Wherever I went with my colleagues, I got wasted. My goal was to get really drunk, to laugh, and to have fun. I thought that living life to the fullest meant getting totally intoxicated every weekend and doing crazy things. I didn't stop to consider that people might not want to follow a leader that was completely drunk all of the time.

It is truly amazing that I am still alive today. I certainly had a guardian angel looking after me. At 22 years old, I didn't know what I didn't know, but looking back, I was so irresponsible. I would drive home for more than an hour from team night drunk on Thursdays. I would act so foolishly around colleagues and other business owners at conferences because I had too much alcohol at the free cocktail hour. I would go to Sun's parties on the weekend and get so drunk that I would fall down or have to sleep there because there was no way they would let me get behind the wheel of the car.

One night, I went out to a club in Boston with my colleague, Sara, and some of her friends. Sara was my closest friend at Maxwell, and we had formed a tight bond, because we started working there on the same day. She lived in the college neighborhood of Allston, near Boston University.

After we returned home from the bar, I went outside on Sara's porch to smoke a cigarette and make a phone call to Walter, who was my fiancé at the time. When I went to go back inside, I realized that someone had locked me out. I tried calling a couple of people who had come out with us that evening, but no one answered. I tried pounding on the sliding glass door, but no one heard me. When I looked inside, everyone was passed out on the sofas and the floor.

What am I going to do? I thought to myself.

I couldn't drive home because my keys were inside my bag in the house. I was also barefoot. It was summertime in Boston, but it was still a bit chilly and definitely not warm enough yet to sleep outside on the porch. I decided to climb over Sara's porch and onto her neighbor's. I looked inside through their glass sliding door. When I looked inside, all I saw were beer cans everywhere.

Good, I thought. This is likely another college house.

I attempted to open the neighbor's sliding glass door, and to my surprise, it was unlocked! I walked into the house quietly and listened carefully, but it seemed that everyone was asleep or not home yet. I quietly snuck through the kitchen to the living room and opened their front door. I walked across the hall and banged on Sara's front door so many times, but no one heard me, because everyone had passed out. I tried calling her and a few other people again, but no one answered.

How is it that no one can hear me banging on the door? I thought. Where am I going to sleep?

I sat down on the floor of the hallway to think. How could they be so drunk that they remembered to lock the porch door and their front door, but forgot that I was out there? (As if I wouldn't do something like that.) Ugh, I was so frustrated, and I wasn't sure what to do.

I decided to go out the front door of the building, making sure it didn't lock behind me, to check to see if my car was open. I had my manual lock 97' blue Chevy Cavalier, and so maybe I had forgotten to lock one of the doors and I could sleep there for the night. As I stepped out on the street of Boston and onto Sara's front walk, I stepped on something sharp. It turned out to be a piece of glass that cut my foot.

"Ow! Oh, man!" I said out loud. My foot was bleeding, and I still had no place to sleep. As I hobbled to my car that was parked down the road, I discovered that I indeed had locked all four doors and there was no way to get into it. Since that was the case, I hobbled back to the apartment building and went back into the entranceway of Sara's building. This time I was sure to step over the pile of glass that I had just stepped on so that I wouldn't cut myself again.

I stood at the entrance of the building and looked right at the door to Sara's apartment. Then I looked left at the neighbor's apartment that I had entered from the back porch. I had no place to sleep, and I was bleeding. To me, I had no other choice, and I decided to enter the neighbor's apartment on the left.

When I entered their apartment, a warm feeling came rushing over me. Again, there was no one to be found, and it was completely quiet. I found a napkin and was able to stop the bleeding on my foot. The adrenaline and the alcohol had left me worn out, and I was exhausted. I laid down on the couch in the living room and pulled the New England Patriots blanket that was draped on the sofa over me. I fell asleep right away.

I woke up the next morning and felt that there were people standing right over me. I decided to keep my eyes closed, but I heard them say the following:

"Who is this girl?"

"Where did she come from?"

"Has anyone seen her before?"

"Did she go out with us last night?"

"Should we call the police?"

"Is this Becca's friend?"

"Is this the girl who hooked up with Tommy?"

Oh, my gosh, the girls who lived there had woken up and found me. I was so embarrassed, but I decided to stay still and pretend I was still sleeping. I was hoping to have woken up before them, but the alcohol had made me sleep past my alarm. Apparently, these girls were just as drunk as my friends, because they didn't remember if I had hung out with them the night before.

Eventually they left me sleeping and went back into their rooms. As soon as I heard the door close, I got up and snuck out the front door. I banged on my friend's door, and to my luck, it was open.

Thank God, I thought. That was so embarrassing.

It turned out that Sara had woken up to go to the bathroom and had seen my texts from the night before about me trying to get into her apartment. So she had unlocked the front door.

"Oh my gosh, Christine! Where were you, I was worried sick?" Sara said.

And so I explained that I had been locked out, cut my foot, and decided to sleep on the neighbor's sofa because the door was open.

Sara could not stop laughing. "Are you serious!?" You slept on the neighbor's couch? I don't even know those girls."

I guess the story was funny from an outsider's perspective, but it could have been really dangerous. I refused to go back to Sara's apartment ever again in fear of running into one of the neighbors. At least they did not call the police on me for breaking and entering.

Monday, at work, Sun came up to me and said, "Seibold, you slept on a stranger's sofa?!" and let out a laugh so strong I couldn't help but smile as my face lit up like a Christmas tree.

LESSONS LEARNED

You are the sum of those who you surround yourself with. Choose friends who are responsible, caring, respectful, and thoughtful. Be careful of your actions, and don't put yourself in dangerous situations. Be conscious of how much you drink so that you do not get out of control. And don't forget to love yourself.

CAPÍTULO QUINCE: HARVARD SHMARVARD

After we passed through the crowd of people and the *huelga*, we found ourselves at the entrance of the university. It used to be an old Tobacco Factory that they turned into the University in 1978. It was also the university I attended when I studied abroad my sophomore and junior years.

We walked through the center towards the big fountain in the middle. Staircases lined both sides of the building, and I reminisced about when I was a student there. We walked into the bar at the University and ordered a café con leche. I remember I used to think it was so cool that my school had a bar in it when I lived there, especially when I was 19. (Oh, the alcohol!)

I started to think about when I studied at Harvard, and how different the two schools were.

I feel very fortunate to have been able to both work and study at Harvard University. I worked for The Harvard School of Public Health, now the Harvard T.H. Chan School of Public Health, for five years of my career. When I moved home from Spain, I started out at Harvard in a temporary position as the assistant to the Director in the Department of Executive and Continuing Education. After the position ended, I left briefly and then was hired back in the same department as a program coordinator. Later, I was promoted to a program manager.

My time working at Harvard was a great experience. It taught me how to manage various projects at one time and work with all different kinds of people from all over the world. In fact, I don't think I would have had the skills or the confidence to be able to run my own business if I had not worked there. I owe a lot to Harvard (thankfully, not in student loans) and would definitely not be where I am today without my time there. That being said, I was completely ready to move on and out of Boston at the end of my five years there.

In my time as a program manager, I was responsible for the logistics and planning of executive education programs for physicians and others who worked in the health field to attend. I would develop and run anywhere from 6-8 programs a year. Apart from logistics, I would work together with the Harvard faculty and program directors to plan the program content and make sure it was executed the way that they liked it.

One particular professor that I worked with had been at Harvard for what seemed like the beginning, when Harvard was founded in 1636. Professor Evan Maddox was an Irish faculty member who ran the top leadership program for physicians in our department. He was well-known for many things, one of them being the most difficult faculty member to work with. Everyone in my department was scared of him, including the directors, and let him get away with horrible things. Everyone just called him Evan, his first name.

One day, as I sat down with my supervisor for our one-on-one meeting, she told me that I was going to get promoted from a program coordinator to a program manager. However, in order to be promoted, there would be one condition. The condition was that I had to take over the programs working with Evan. My heart and my head sank. The excitement that I felt when I was told of my promotion suddenly turned into fear. I had already worked with Evan for a year as a coordinator filtering through applications for the program, and he made my blood boil. He really tested my patience.

At first sight, Evan appeared to be a polite Irish gentleman. He had a stern, tough side to him, and he would not stop at anything until he got what he wanted. He always fought to get his way, or he would take up the situation with the dean of the university. He always ended up winning and getting what he wanted. There is definitely something about Harvard and having seniority. It was like an unwritten rule. I had heard of numerous stories from the past of him mistreating people and being disrespectful and rude. Naturally, I was scared that he would be the same way with me and there would be nothing I could do about it if I wanted to keep my job.

He was so particular about so many things. For example, he would refuse to use email. Yes, my people, in 2016, Evan Maddox claimed he did not know how to use email and that he didn't even have email at home, even though we knew he did. Every faculty member at Harvard was automatically assigned an email address, so he had to have one. He just chose not to use it. Since Evan did not use email, any correspondence or communication with him had to be done via the telephone or fax. That's right. The FAX machine. The fax machine that sat in our manager's office did not even work correctly and half of the time the faxes were not delivered or received.

Anyone in our office who worked with Evan was forced to set up a fax system on their computers called e-fax, so that they would get an email anytime they received a fax from him. The program allowed us to see a picture of the document.

I can just hear him calling my desk now, in his old Irish accent, saying "Hello, Christine, did you receive my fax?" Needless to say, Evan loved paper.

The leadership course that he directed was a very intense two-week program that always filled up with 48-50 physicians.

Along with those two weeks came a lot of case studies and articles. In order to attend, you had to apply and be accepted into the program. It was my job to receive all of the applications and submit them to Evan for review. I was also in charge of organizing all of the course materials and having all of the cases and readings printed out into binders in the order that Evan wanted. At registration, on the first day of the program, each physician would receive three huge binders full of materials. Needless to say, it was a lot of paper.

I was always so terrified on the first day of the program each year. It was like a big test that I had prepared for, for six months. Evan was definitely a man of systems, and everything had to be the way and the order that he liked it. He would come strolling into the Colonnade Hotel with his Irish hat, suitcoat, and briefcase. Just as he was a man of habit and order, he always wore the same thing on the first day of the program.

One year, the printing company that created our binders had a new employee, and they completely messed up the materials in the binders. However we didn't notice until the morning of the start of the program when we went to set up. I pictured Evan walking in with his suitcoat and hat with my head on a platter. I had seen Evan get upset before with other people, and I didn't want this to be the first time with me.

Evan was known for humiliating people in public. Behind closed doors, he had called my colleague an idiot amongst other names and seemed to like to put people down to make sure everyone knew he was the boss and in control. He even went after the director of our department, so I knew he had no trouble coming for me.

Eventually, the day came when I made a "huge mistake" during the program. I think I forgot to put out a set of handouts during the break of the program because I was helping out one of the participants. Evan came into the office and made it quite clear how disappointed and upset he was with me.

Needless to say, Evan was a very persistent man, and very strong-willed. He did what he needed to do in order to get what he wanted. He was very proud, a bit arrogant, and would stop at nothing until things were the way he wanted. Thankfully, he lived outside of Boston, so he was not constantly running into the office. However he would visit in person about once a week to pick up any mail and paper applications that had arrived. However, since he lived outside of the city and was not at the school every day, he would call… and he would call me a lot.

At one point, I felt like I was spending the whole day on the phone with Evan, and I could not get anything else done. I had 6 other programs that I was in charge of planning, which meant 6 other program directors and faculty that I had to manage. I could not do that with Evan calling me every few minutes with a request, an order, a job, a fax, or something else that he needed. It got to the point that I felt like my paycheck was coming from Evan Maddox, and not Harvard University, and I didn't like it.

In a one-on-one meeting with my manager, I expressed my frustration and concern. Clearly, I was less than excited to be Evan Maddox's work horse, or so I felt, but the answer was always, "There is not really much I can do." That was always the answer because everyone was afraid of him, not because there wasn't anything that could be done. No one had the guts to stand up to him and say no. No one had the guts to set any boundaries with him. After various frustrating meetings like this, my manager was finally able to get support from the directors of the department to back her up. She told me I had the right to say no to some things that he requested, that I could demand that I needed time to complete different requests, and that I could not answer the phone when he called all of the time.

And so that is what I started to do. It seemed strange, as I would see his number pop up on my caller ID, but I was in the middle of something else and did not want to stop. I was always tempted to answer it, but I didn't pick up. I felt like I was doing something sinful, and my heart would race. Then he would call again a few minutes later. He would call and call again and leave message after message. Then he would get mad, and he would call my manager to tell her I wasn't picking up. He wasn't used to not getting his way.

Thankfully, my manager had a meeting with him to explain that I had other work to do and that I could not just be his slave. This made him even angrier. I didn't want him to get mad at me, but at the same time, I didn't want him bothering me all day every day. Either way, it was a lose-lose situation.

I am happy to say that I was there the day that Evan was "fired" from Harvard. Or we can say, he was forced into retirement. It definitely was one of the best days in my five years there. I never thought that day would come, but it did. They had built up a case against him for years, and they were finally able to present to the dean the reasons why now was a good time for Evan to "retire." The dean finally agreed, and he went with it. I think at that point the dean was just sick and tired of people coming and complaining about Evan, or Evan going to him to complain when he didn't get his way, and he finally had had enough.

There was definitely a sense of freedom from not having Evan around anymore. I didn't have to work in fear of making a mistake and making everything perfect the way he wanted. I must say, Evan did make me a better proofreader. I learned the hard way by handing in documents to him that had not been proofread or full of mistakes.

They ended up hiring my favorite faculty member to take his place, and I was super excited to work with her. She later ended up being my advisor for my master's thesis. The first year that she took over the programs, we ran them the same way that we did when Evan was the director so she could see how the programs were laid out. She was in shock at some of the things my colleague and I told her about Evan and how the program was handled. The good news was that she was quite open, and the best thing of all was that she used email!

The day I got rid of the e-fax program I had a little celebration. I did a little dance at my desk. No more running to the fax machine to send faxes and no more receiving faxes into my email with handwritten notes that I could barely read. The wrath of Evan was over, and I could not be happier.

LESSONS LEARNED

It is important to set boundaries with those that you work with. It is best to set guidelines or rules from the beginning for others to adapt to and follow. Don't let anyone mistreat you at your workplace. Say no to people and projects that do not feel right. We teach others how we want to be treated, so remember to respect and love yourself, and others will show you the respect and love back.

CAPÍTULO DIESISÉIS: SARA BROWN

After our *café con leche* at the bar, we walked through the rest of the University. Walking through the patio in the open air with students passing by made me think of my time on campus at my undergraduate college in Albany, New York.

I attended the College of Saint Rose, a small private school of about 4,000 undergraduates and 1,000 graduate students. I never thought that I would go to a city that was colder and where it snowed more than in Boston. However, as I mentioned previously, I went to Albany for school to be closer to my boyfriend Earl of three years at the time, which as you know, did not end up working out.

Albany didn't have much that was attractive about it, with its trashy downtown and boring architecture. Still to this day, I cannot figure out why it is the capital of New York, and why New York City isn't. Albany was known as a big party city due to the 31 universities that were in its 25-mile radius, which fit in perfectly with my drinking and party lifestyle at the time. It often reminded me of Worcester, Massachusetts, back home where I grew up.

One thing about Albany was that everyone had a fake ID. The New York State license was made to be fake. My license from Massachusetts was a hard laminated plastic. The New York license was more like a thicker paper or cardboard that was not shiny or laminated and allowed for people to write on it. The letters and numbers were written in red and green. Saint Rose was a school of the arts, and so one way that the art major students would make money on the side was by charging a fee to change someone's birthdate on their license to make them 21. That way they could go out and buy alcohol or go to clubs and drink. While I saw some pretty convincing fake IDs, or IDs that had their dates changed, the bars in the area also knew that almost everyone who went there was lying about their age and usually would not turn you away from entering.

Naturally, due to my obsession with alcohol and drinking, I had to get my hands on one of those IDs.

"Here, take it," my friend Andrea said as she pushed the ID in my face.

She had come to visit me in my dorm room since she lived just down the hall. I don't even remember how or where she got the ID, but she already had one and was offering this one to me, so I took it. I looked at the information on the license to see if it was a match:

*Name: Sara Brown - Check.

*Height: 5'9" - Check.

*Eye Color: Green – Well, blue is close enough to green, I thought. - Check.

*Photo: She had long straight dirty blonde hair like me, but her face was much thinner. *I can make it work,* I thought. *I'm going to lose those 50 pounds this year anyway.* - Check.

*Age: Oh, man, she was born in 1978, I thought. My birthday is in 1982, but I guess it is close enough. I can pass for a 23-year-old, right? That's ok, I thought. This will definitely do. - Check.

And there I was, 19 years old, and just like that, I had my first fake ID. I took the ID from Andrea and just prayed that I didn't lose it some drunken night or have it taken away from me from a bouncer who was in a bad mood.

Those were the good old days. I remember the bars in the area like it was yesterday. Pauley's, The Post, The Washington Tavern, and The Raven always had drink specials for the college students in the area. They were all within walking distance of our campus.

On Wednesdays, the Tavern had buy-one/get-one free beers. On Thursdays, Pauley's had 25 cent cups of beer until 11 p.m. (my favorite), so we would go there early around 9 p.m. when it wasn't too busy yet. On Fridays, The Post gave you a free pitcher of beer if you arrived before 10 p.m.. On Saturdays, we would usually venture further downtown to the main street of bars and try to get into those with our IDs. It was always a 50/50 chance with a fake ID downtown because the bars were more regulated. It depended on if you knew the guy who was working at the door. But at least if the bouncers downtown suspected you were not 21, they wouldn't take your ID.

They would just give it back to you and say, "Sorry, we can't let you in."

But the other bars did not really care. They just cared about making money.

One weekend, Patty came to visit me from Worcester, and we somehow managed to get her a fake ID to go out. We thought The Post was our best chance because they were usually the most lenient. The Post would let anyone in, or so we thought. Patty was about 5'2" with heels on and was very petite. Even to this day, she looks about 10 years younger than her real age.

We got dressed and walked down the street about a half of a mile to The Post. Patty and I had been best friends since high school, and we were both giddy and excited that she was visiting.

When we arrived at the door of the bar, I felt a sense of relief because I had seen the bouncer a million times before. He looked at Patty and then looked at her ID, and then looked at Patty and then looked at the ID.

To our surprise, he said, "Sorry, ladies, not tonight." And he turned us away.

I could not believe it! He told Patty he did not believe she was 21. Frustrated and puzzled about what we were going to do for the evening, we sadly walked home to my dorm to try to figure out alternate plans.

After we concluded that there was really nothing else going on on-campus, we decided we would change our clothes, and give The Post another try. When we returned the second time, there was a different guy at the door, and he let us in! Woohoo! Our excitement that had faded away from being turned down the first time quickly returned as we entered the bar with blaring music. We thought we were slick, and we joked about my drunk alter ego "Sara Brown." Patty and I danced and drank the night away and had so much fun together, as always.

My dorm room during my freshman year of college was a forced triple. That meant that it was supposed to be a double, but due to high enrollment, they had turned it into a triple because there was no other place to put the freshmen students. Needless to say, it was extremely cramped with an extra bed, dresser, and desk. My roommates were Cassidy, a gorgeous, well-off New Yorker who was recruited to play soccer at my college, and Dawn, a very petite, rather snobby well-off local who was a bit lost and hadn't decided what to study yet. She was always sad and missing her family who lived twenty minutes away. From day one, I got along much better with Cassidy, who was a tomboy and was always very kind to me. She liked to party and go out, whereas Dawn was more of a homebody, but would go out occasionally.

By now we have already established that I did not do the most honorable things when I got drunk, especially in college. I went through a period where I wanted to decorate my room with college memorabilia. But I was a college student and didn't have money to buy the memorabilia, so I got into the habit of stealing it from the bars. I would carry a big purse out with me and take things home. Sometimes it was the glass that my beer was in with the logo from the bar. Other times it was something from the counter of the bar, and oftentimes it was a decoration or sign. I got such a high from being sneaky and taking things home. My friends started calling me "Stealing Sara" (named after Sara Brown), but they would laugh and go along with it. Everyone thought the things that I would take were hilarious, and occasionally Cassidy would join in and take something with me. It soon became a game.

Now, I've always had a rather strong personality. I don't necessarily like being the center of attention, but when I was drunk, my personality would get even bigger. I definitely liked the attention. I mean, I was Sara Brown, right? I was always searching for a way to be loved and accepted, and so I think my crazy actions were a way for me to get attention and be "loved by others."

I remember when Cassidy was laughing with me, she would say, "I friggin love you girl!" and so that was some kind of love, right?

By the end of my freshman year, I had collected a lot of bar memorabilia. I had so much that I was really running out of room to put it (especially in the forced triple dorm room). I don't know what changed in me when I got to college to give me a sense of entitlement to take these objects and think that it was okay to steal. That was definitely not the way I was raised. I decided that it was Sara Brown's fault.

Eventually I lost my fake ID, so I couldn't go out to bars, just house parties. It didn't make too much of a difference because I ended up leaving New York to study abroad in Spain my sophomore year and the drinking age there is 18, so I didn't need a fake ID. When I came back from Spain, I only had a few months before I turned 21, so I never got a new fake ID. Sara Brown was gone, but her evil twin remained inside of me, even without the ID for many years to come.

LESSONS LEARNED

Don't take what is not yours. Stealing to get others to accept and like you is not the way to live. Drinking in excess will often cause you to behave in ways that you would not normally behave. Be honest, be kind, and love yourself.

CAPÍTULO DIECISIETE: PUSH, PUSH, SHOVE, SHOVE

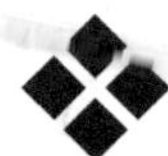

As we stepped outside of the university, I could feel the Seville sun beating down on my face. The familiar, warm feeling made me happy inside and filled me with energy. Oh, how much I loved the sun! As we stepped onto the sidewalk about to cross the street, a Chinese tour bus flew right past us. Seeing the Chinese tour bus brought me back to my Europe trip with my dad and our encounter with a big group of Chinese tourists in Russia.

The day that I decided to leave Ahmed, was also the day that I went on a trip with my dad to Europe. I had originally planned to meet Ahmed in Morocco to spend time with his family. After Morocco, we had planned to travel for two weeks to different countries in Europe. However, after discovering the secret Facebook page and him lunging at me, there was no way that I was going to go anywhere with him.

But, I still wanted to go away and was hoping to have something like an *Eat, Pray, Love* experience. I had already taken the vacation time from work and the tickets were non-refundable, so I decided to plan a new trip to go to different places without Ahmed. I needed some time away to clear my head and figure out what the next steps were going to be in my life after being a divorced woman twice at the age of 33.

Naturally, my parents were worried about me and my emotional state after the breakup, and so my dad offered to come with me on the trip so I didn't have to go alone. I always wish that the United States had a transportation system and cheap airlines just like Europe does. Once you get over there, it is easy and inexpensive to travel around.

And so off we went. My dad met me in Madrid, and we went to Stockholm, Sweden, Copenhagen, Denmark, and Helsinki, Finland. The style of the Scandinavian countries was very different from the rest of Europe. They were quite beautiful with the square, colorful architecture, their tin roofs, lots of bicycles, and everything was very organized. However, they were also quite expensive as well.

My dad was a trooper and stayed in hostels or small inns with me. Our accommodations were reserved last-minute due to the circumstances and changes of the trip. My budget was low, especially since I had already lost a good chunk of money from the trip that I had planned with Ahmed. It was also July, which was vacation prime time for tourists, especially in Scandinavia, and so everything was expensive.

After Scandinavia, we took an overnight ferry from Finland to St. Petersburg, Russia. The Russian government has a rule for Americans that allows you to enter the country without a visa if you promise to stay for less than 72 hours, so we found a tour and that is exactly what we did.

St. Petersburg was such a beautiful city. It was much more advanced and cleaner than I expected. I was expecting a Cold War, gloomy, depressed atmosphere, but it was the complete opposite.

Some days on the trip I was an emotional mess and questioning whether I had made the right decision to leave

Ahmed. Part of me could not really enjoy the new countries too much because I felt so sad, and my head was spinning. Ahmed had tried contacting me non-stop for the first few days, which caused me to block him from different numbers and create a whole new email address. There were times that I doubted my decision. But my mind kept going back to that horrible night when my sister discovered the Facebook page with naked women and that reminded me that I had made the right decision and that he would not change.

I was also a bit scared about the unknown and what my life would be like once I returned to Boston. But my dad reassured me that I had made the right decision, and he was there to listen to me, hug me when I cried, and share stories of his own. We had a great time together, and I really enjoyed his company. I didn't want the time to end.

Some of my favorite memories with my dad include having breakfast at the Espresso Café (a chain restaurant that we went to in each Scandinavian country), watching my dad take a shot of Russian vodka, picking out a necklace at the open market in Finland that was made from their labradorite stone, and trying ice cream from all of the different countries.

I also remember him sharing with me a beautiful story at dinner one evening on our way to Russia. He shared with me how much he loved my mom unconditionally, how he would do anything for her, and how he wanted my sisters and I to find that same kind of love. That one had us both sobbing.

I looked at him in awe and was amazed that he had been with my mom for 45 years at that point. I sat there and felt the gratitude that I had for them, for their unending support for me. I prayed that someday God would find an amazing man like my father, who was meant for me, to truly love me unconditionally, just as I am. I often wondered if that was possible and if I would ever get married again.

As we waited in line in St. Petersburg to get onto the cruise ship to go back to Finland, I couldn't help but notice that the majority of the passengers on the ship were Chinese. I didn't think anything of it until the next morning when we arrived back in Finland. They had directed everyone on the ship to come with our luggage to the main lobby to wait for the ship to dock so that we could get off. What we had learned from getting off of the ship in Russia was that they were only allowing us to leave from one exit door of the ship.

The lobby started to fill up quickly with all of the passengers who were eager to get off of the boat. Soon the room was very full and could not hold any more people. The elevator doors would open with people arriving from upstairs and there was no place to let them off of the elevator. There must have been 200-300 people with their luggage in that room. Everyone seemed very tense and eager to get off of the boat, and I had the feeling that something was going to happen. We had docked, but for some reason, it seemed to take forever to open the doors and we didn't know why.

As soon as they opened the exit door, everyone started pushing, and the atmosphere turned quite chaotic. I didn't understand what the reason was to push. Everyone was going to get off, and it was only 7 in the morning, so what was the rush?

My dad and I held back and let everyone go in front of us. I took out my iPhone and started filming the scene. Right after I started filming, one of the Chinese couples pushed an older German man and his wife and his wife fell down on the ground. He got extremely angry and screamed at them in German. This caused the pushing to slow down a bit, but soon after, everyone was pushing again.

I have nothing against the Chinese culture, but I have traveled to various countries and have seen the pushing with

Chinese people before. We had also seen it in line at the museum in Russia the day before.

Pushing does not get you anywhere faster, and it can cause people to get injured. I have had experiences in other countries with Chinese people and boundaries around personal space, and it is very frustrating to encounter. It must be a cultural thing. Anyway, this time, it was quite a funny scene and made me feel like I was in a movie.

My dad and I were one of the last ones to get off of the ship. Needless to say, our trip to Russia was unforgettable and memorable. We spent another day in Helsinki and then my Dad left me to go back to Boston. He had to go back to work, and I headed on to Estonia and Greece on my own. I am so grateful for the experiences we had together, for all of the laughs and cries and, most importantly, the time.

The trip was very special to me, and it was the first time that I had gone anywhere just with my dad. I changed inside, and for the first time in a long time, I had some hope when I returned to Boston and to work at the end of the three-week trip. It is definitely a time that I will never forget and will always hold dear to my heart.

LESSONS LEARNED

Respect people and their space. There is no need to push anywhere for any reason, especially in large groups. Different cultures react differently in large crowds, especially in unknown places. When you are going through tough times, surround yourself with those who love you. It is ok to ask for help. Protect yourself, put your safety first, take care of yourself, and love yourself.

CAPÍTULO DIECIOCHO: PIZZA PIZZA

Every time I leave Seville, I cry. It is the only other place in the world that feels like home to me. The way the culture is laid back, the food is so fresh and tasty, the beauty of the architecture, the flamenco, the way they value family and enjoy life, all aligns with what I love in life.

Sadly, our trip was coming to an end, and as usual, I did not want to leave. We left the university, crossed the street, and headed into the Maria Luisa Park one more time.

We strolled around the *Plaza de España* before we headed back to the hotel. We walked down Constitution Avenue in the center and passed by the Cathedral, tourist shops, restaurants, street entertainers, flamenco dancers, and the main post office one more time. No matter how many times I walk by, the old Moorish architecture leaves me breathless with its beautiful shapes, designs, and colors. When the sun shines down on the buildings, it shows the artistry and talent of the Moorish architecture that was built back in the 700s.

We were leaving Seville that evening and taking the fast Ave train up to Madrid. The main purpose for stopping there was to see my favorite singer in concert, Enrique Iglesias. It had been over five years since Enrique had sang a concert in his native city of Madrid, and I was super excited that we were going to be there at the same time. He was such a good performer with amazing energy and pretty easy on the eye too. I also wanted to show Anderson the capital city of Spain.

When we arrived back at the hotel, we grabbed a quick snack and packed up our suitcases. A part of me wondered when we were going to be back here together. *Would we be able to return to Seville to live here in the near future? Did Anderson even like Spain that much?* Apart from the first day, we hadn't really discussed his like or dislike for it.

We called an Uber to take us to Santa Justa, the train station. Anderson bought our tickets from the ticket booth, and as he turned around, he could see my eyes were welling up with tears.

"We are going to be back soon, love. Don't worry." He knew me so well. There was just something so special and magical about Seville that made me never want to leave.

We walked to the platform, boarded the train, and found our seats. We stored our suitcases and put our bags above us. As we sat down, I could smell a fresh pizza. *Mmmmm* I thought to myself. *I could go for one of those right about now.*

I looked over at the couple in the seats across from us and saw that they had bought a pizza for the trip. As the man brought a piece to his mouth, the sauce splattered all over his shirt. I covered my mouth so I wouldn't laugh out loud at him. As the man grabbed a napkin and began to wipe off the sauce, it made me have flashbacks to a crazy Brazilian party that I went to with my cousin Ana.

By this point in the book, you may have gathered that I am a very international person. My only American boyfriend was Earl, and then I dated a Colombian, a Brazilian, a Dominican, and the list just grows more international from there.

There was a group of Brazilians that I used to hang out with who lived outside of Boston who really knew how to enjoy life. In fact, it was through that group of friends that I met Walter. Massachusetts is flooded with Brazilians, most of them from the state of Minas Gerais. In the 1980s, there was a big immigration of Brazilians to Massachusetts and many families migrated from small Brazilian towns and settled in the Northeast.

This particular group of friends that we had were all from the same small town, and so they knew each other very well since they grew up together. Brazilians love their *churrascos*, or barbecues, and they love cold beer and *cachaça* (as we established in Chapter 7).

My cousin Ana and I have always been very close. She grew up on Long Island and is just a couple of years older than me. Often, she would drive up to Massachusetts to visit me, and we would go visit the Brazilians when they had a party. We would have such a good time and have the greatest conversations. We both trust each other a lot and will go to the grave with some of our secrets.

One weekend, Ana came to visit, and we attended a Brazilian party. Ana had a crush on Felipe, my boyfriend Leo's roommate at the time. There is something attractive about working hard, but then knowing how to leave work behind and just laugh and tell stories, whip out the guitar to sing, and just have a good time with some beers and good food. Americans have a hard time disconnecting from work sometimes, so I admire the Brazilian culture for their ability to do so.

We arrived at the party around 9 p.m., and there were already about 15 people there. The house was super small, and four people lived in the one-bedroom home. It was more like a garage with a living room, kitchen, and a bedroom in the back that had two bunk beds. Another truth about many Brazilians is that they often live together in a rather cramped lifestyle to keep the rent low, at least in the beginning, when they first arrive in the country.

The party was super fun with about 20 plus people (mostly Brazilian men) crammed into the small living room. The

Brazilians were all happy to see my cousin Ana again, and they welcomed us with open arms. I looked around, and everyone was dancing, drinking, passing around Brazilian barbecue and pizza, yelling and telling stories, and having a great time.

At one point, Leo and I started arguing about something. I decided I needed some fresh air and went to look for Ana, but she was nowhere to be found. I walked through the rooms of the house, and asked some of the guys at the party, but they did not know where she was. I noticed Felipe was missing too, so I checked with Leo. He told me that Ana and Felipe had run out to the gas station to get gas.

That is kind of weird, I thought. *Who needs gas on a Friday night at 1 a.m.?* But, I didn't think too much of it and went back to listening to a funny story in the group.

Another hour went by, and Ana and Felipe still had not returned. I could not find my bag with my cell phone, so Leo called Felipe's phone, and there was no answer. It just rang and rang. He kept trying, but it just went to his voicemail.

"I hope they are okay," I said to Leo. "I am getting worried. It is almost 2:30 a.m." Leo nodded his head in agreement as he took another sip of his drink. We were both too drunk to try to drive anywhere to go and find them.

The party started to die down around 5 a.m. Some people left, and others passed out on the floor. I looked around, and the house was such a mess. Besides it being a total bachelor pad, there was pizza everywhere, beer cans and cups, spilled drinks on the tables, empty liquor bottles, and even towels and clothes sprawled throughout the home. One of the guys who lived there thought it was a good idea to have a fashion show at around 3 a.m., and had left his clothes everywhere.

There was no sign of Ana, and I was super worried. I was also super drunk and ended up passing out with Leo in one of the beds in the back room. We had been sleeping for about two hours when there was a loud noise in the front of the house. Someone had been banging on the front door, and so one of the Brazilians who had passed out in the living room opened it. The guy who opened the door was Samuel, and he was covered in pizza and had sauce all over his face and shirt. To everyone's surprise, it was my father who had been making the noise! In my dad's broken Spanish/Portuguese that he knew, he told Samuel that he was looking for Christine.

Samuel let my dad in the living room, and my dad stared at him up and down and just said *"Vocé gosta da pizza, eh?"* (You like pizza eh?)

Samuel just smiled and came to the back of the home where Leo and I were sleeping and woke us up to tell us that MY DAD WAS IN THE LIVING ROOM!

I couldn't believe what he was saying, and I thought I hadn't heard him correctly. *How did my dad even know where I was? I* looked around the room and did not see Ana or Felipe. *What was my dad going to say when he asked where Ana was? How was I going to tell him that I didn't know where she went?* All of these thoughts flooded my head, and my heart started beating fast. I walked into the living room where my dad was standing in the middle of four other Brazilians passed out on the floor. I, myself, was still quite drunk.

"Morning," my dad said in a stern voice. "Looks like some party you guys had here last night." He stared down at the guys passed out on the floor and then at Samuel, who my dad insisted on calling "Pizza Face." I just nodded my head and squinted my eyes as they adjusted to the sunlight that was beaming through the window.

My dad continued, "So I received a call at 6 a.m. this morning from the Bolton Police Department. Felipe is in jail and Ana is waiting for us at the police station."

"WHAT?!" I said as I immediately went from drunk to sober. "Are they ok?" I asked. "Why are they in jail?"

My dad went on to explain that the police said that they came across Felipe's car that was parked on the side of the road. The police tapped on the window to see if they were ok and asked Felipe for this license. Felipe did not have a license, and he also had some unpaid parking tickets, so they took him away to spend the night in jail. Ana had a driver's license, but she did not know how to drive a stick shift, so she could not drive Felipe's car home, and it was towed.

Since she had no other options, the cop took Ana down to the same station where Felipe was in jail.

I could not believe what I was hearing! I was relieved that they were both safe though. What happened to getting a phone call? I explained to my dad that Leo had tried calling Felipe, and he didn't answer, and I couldn't find my phone, so I didn't know where they had gone. Ana reminded me later that my phone was in my purse that she had put in the car, which is why I couldn't find it.

I grabbed my things, kissed Leo goodbye, and went with my dad to pick up Ana and Felipe from the police station. When I got into the car, my mother was also there. *Oh, great. No I am really in trouble.*

My dad bailed Felipe out, and he promised that he would show up to his court date so my dad would get his bond money returned. Ana was pretty quiet and just kept her head down. I could tell she was embarrassed as the four of us climbed into the car in silence.

We stopped at the tow lot to get Felipe's car out. Since Felipe did not have a license, my dad used his and drove Felipe's car back to where the party had been. *My dad is such a champ,* I thought. My parents were pretty cool about the whole thing. I made sure to tell them later. We followed behind him, and Felipe thanked my parents over and over for their help.

When my dad got back in the car to drive us home, Ana said, "I'm sorry, Uncle Mike and Aunt Rosemary. I didn't mean for any of this to happen. Thank you for coming to get us."

My dad said, "Sure, Ana. I am just happy that everyone is safe."

The three of us drove home in silence. As we approached our home, my dad said, "What is up with Pizza Face? He had pizza all over his face and his clothes."

Ana and I just looked at each other and burst out laughing.

LESSONS LEARNED

Life is a party, but party with caution. Excessive drinking can cause you to do things that are out of character or that put you in danger. You can also get lost and end up in places that you do not want to be. Drinking can have serious health effects on you later in life. You can also end up scaring your loved ones when you put yourself in dangerous situations. Take care of yourself, take care of your health, and don't forget to love yourself.

CAPÍTULO DIECINUEVE: FIGHT IN FLIGHT

Anderson and I arrived in Madrid at around midnight and took an Uber to our hotel. We were just staying there for two nights and then would be heading to Israel for the second part of our trip. Madrid was beautifully decorated with Christmas lights throughout the streets. The plazas and alleys were filled with people outside in the warm winter evening walking and enjoying the beautiful Christmas decorations.

The next day, I took Anderson to the famous Plaza Mayor, the Castle, and the city center, and then we headed back to the hotel to get ready for the Enrique Iglesias concert. We must have walked 10 miles.

The concert was AMAZING. I will never forget it. I bought the tickets as a birthday present to myself, and it was the first time ever that I had standing floor seats for the show. Enrique did not disappoint, and we got so close to him at one point that we could almost touch him. That was my third Enrique Iglesias concert, and by far, it was the best. We grabbed a late dinner after the concert and took it home to eat in the nice, warm hotel room. It was hard to admit that our Spain leg of the trip was over. At least we ended it with a bang!

The next morning, we headed out early to go to the airport. As soon as we got on the metro, my eyes filled with tears (again). It was not a foreign event to me, because the uncertainty of the next time that I would return to Spain always brought me a sense of sadness.

Although the trip was good overall, it wasn't what I had expected. I wanted Anderson to fall in love with Seville and have a passion for it as much as I do, but I wasn't sure that he did. Perhaps memories of living with Ahmed and the flashbacks of the unhappiness that I felt when I was there with him affected my mood a bit. I felt a bit strange, and Anderson did not seem to experience the same excitement for the city that I have every time I go.

As I looked over at him on the train, he leaned in and gave me a hug. He knows me so well and almost always knows what I am thinking without me saying anything. As we approached the airport and went through security, I composed myself and got excited again because the second part of our trip was beginning. We were leaving Spain and heading to Israel.

I had worked on a project in Israel for my master's thesis at Harvard. The leader from the same organization that I worked with for my thesis was writing a book and asked me to write a chapter. Since we were already in Europe, we decided to go to Israel after that so I could do the interviews that were necessary for my chapter in the book.

We left Madrid and had a layover in Turkey. Shortly after we arrived, we were informed that our flight was delayed. As we headed downstairs to our gate, we heard a bunch of women yelling in Arabic. We looked down the stairs, and there were four older women yelling in a panic about something below us. As we arrived at our gate, it became clear to us that they were on our flight, along with a group of about 30 other older Muslim women. All of them were dressed in the traditional Muslim hijab, and they seemed to be anxious about something. We didn't really know what was going on, but we went through a second security check and waited for our flight to start boarding.

Our flight was the kind that required us to take a shuttle to transport us to board from the runway. As the shuttle pulled up, you would have thought that there was free money on it. Everyone got up at once and started bolting towards the door. *Why was everyone in such a hurry?* I thought.

Anderson and I got up and got in the line, only to be cut by a group of these women and their families. Cutting lines is a pet peeve of mind, but I let it pass as it was clear that all these women were together and it was late in the evening. As the line moved forward, more and more of them would just push their way through and cut in front of us. *It must be a cultural thing,* I thought.

It was frustrating, but we let it slide since we were taught to respect our elders. There was a clear language barrier and misunderstanding with these women and the Turkish Airlines workers. The women didn't know how to respond to the security people, and the Turkish Airlines attendants did not know how to communicate with them in Arabic. All I know is there was a lot of shouting and yelling and confusion going on. Some of them were having their bags taken, some of them did not have the right tickets, and none of them knew how to respond.

As you can imagine, a one-hour delay soon turned into a two-hour delay with all the confusion. When we finally boarded the airplane, we observed that most of the women had difficulty reading English numbers, and therefore they could not find their correct seats. Many of them just sat where they wanted, which in turn caused confusion when the person whose seat they were sitting in came on board.

Others just stood in the middle of the aisle blocking people who couldn't get by. Since most of them were older in age, lifting up their suitcases was quite difficult. Since they did not know how to communicate this, many of them decided to leave their carry-ons in the middle of the aisle. Needless to say, the situation was pure chaos.

Do none of the flight attendants on a flight from Turkey to Israel really not speak Arabic? I thought to myself. I couldn't believe it.

Each of the flight attendants tried their hardest to communicate with the women, but the women didn't understand, nor did they seem to care. Each minute that passed would be followed by a flight attendant coming down the aisle rolling one of their suitcases. Either there wasn't room, or they didn't fit above. This chaos continued for about 30 minutes.

Then out of nowhere, a younger man and woman got up and headed towards the front of the plane. The young man went outside on the steps of the plane on his cell phone and stood at the top of the boarding stairs. Meanwhile, the young woman was yelling at the flight attendant in a furious manner in English. The flight attendant closed the curtain at the front of the airplane as the two continued to yell at each other. This fight went on for about 10-15 minutes. I could not hear everything, but I think the passenger was trying to convince the flight attendant to wait for her father to board the plane who was late for the flight.

Why is this flight attendant allowing this man and woman to be on the phone on the steps of the airplane and arguing with her? I thought. Why is she letting this happen? She is in charge, I thought.

The whole scene was absolutely crazy. Half of the flight attendants were dealing with the women and their luggage and trying to find their correct seats, and the other was in the front arguing with the man and woman about God knows what.

After about 45 minutes of this madness, what proceeded to happen next was that people wanted to change their seats to whatever seats were unoccupied. A man plopped himself in the row of empty seats behind us. He was very loud and placed himself there so he could be close to his friends. As soon as he sat down, he would not stop talking and was basically yelling. He must have been a comedian or something because every time he spoke, his friends would crack up laughing. He was speaking in Arabic, so we didn't understand what he was saying, but it reminded me of young boys from middle school.

The man proceeded to talk all through the captain's introduction, and the safety demonstration, until one of the male flight attendants finally said to him in a stern voice, "Sir, please be quiet!"

That worked for about 5 minutes and then he started talking loudly again. As the plane moved to take off, I heard the man speaking to someone on the phone. I looked at Anderson and said, "Is he on the phone right now? Are you kidding me?"

And sure enough, he was speaking on the phone to a woman on speaker phone all the way until we were flying in the air. We were only in row 3, so I couldn't understand why the flight attendant didn't hear him, but she was already in her seat buckled in at that point, so she probably just let it slide. She likely did not want to deal with him, as she had dealt with the chaos before, and the journey had just begun.

Needless to say, the man continued his jokes and spoke loudly throughout the whole flight. Anderson kept turning around and looking at him and giving him dirty looks, but he clearly did not care that he was being disruptive late at night. At one point, he finally had fallen asleep, except the seatbelt sign came on due to turbulence, and the crew woke him up to put his seatbelt on. He subsequently started yelling again.

How rude and disrespectful, I thought. *It is 11:30 p.m., and some people are trying to sleep and relax.* I should have turned around and said something to the man, but I could tell by his demeanor and the way that he spoke that he was one of those men who thought he was above the law and could do whatever he wanted. If he didn't listen to the flight attendants, why would he listen to me? I feared starting another fight on the plane for the Turkish attendants to deal with, so I kept my mouth closed.

When we arrived in Israel, it was 12:30 a.m. We got off of the plane and followed the signs for immigration. *Thank God the line is not too long,* I thought to myself. We still had an hour drive to Jerusalem once we left the airport. The first time I visited Israel was when I was writing my thesis. There was a flood of people who arrived at the same time, and it took two hours to go through immigration.

The immigration lines were divided into sections, so you got to choose which section you wanted to wait in. As we waited in line, the obnoxious man who sat behind us on the plane was impatiently waiting in the line next to ours. Whoever had gone in front of him was getting asked a lot of questions by the officer and had to show documents. It was taking longer than he liked as he stood there huffing and puffing and sighing.

The people in our line in front of us finished their turn, and as they were leaving, the man from the plane started to walk forward like it was his turn because he didn't want to wait any longer in his line.

Ooooooooohhhhhh noooooooo, I thought. You just kept me awake the entire plane ride yelling loud absurd things and now you want to cut me in line. No way! I thought. As I mentioned before, cutting the line was a HUGE pet peeve of mine and I had had enough of him.

"Excuse me, sir!" I said in a loud, stern voice. He kept walking. "Excuse me, sir," I said a second time, even louder. He stopped and turned around. "This is our line," I said as I pointed to our row.

"Oh, sorry, sorry," he replied with his strong accent as he lifted his hands up as if he was innocent. Anderson and I walked forward toward the guard for our turn.

I felt a little scared as my heart was pounding, but I mostly felt proud. I wasn't going to let him get away with treating people however he wanted. You could tell that it was rare that anyone stood up to him or challenged him with anything. Besides, we had already been cut in line all night by the group of women, so it was our turn to stand up for ourselves.

As we picked up our luggage and got into our taxi, the crazy flight that had just taken place passed through my mind. No boundaries with the flight attendants, no boundaries with the women who cut all the lines, and no boundaries with the man sitting behind us who was yelling the whole flight and wanted to cut us in line.

LESSONS LEARNED

Stand up for yourself. Don't be afraid to hold your ground. Even if cultures have different rules about lines and boundaries, don't be afraid to speak up. Be safe when traveling to new countries, be aware of your surroundings, and don't forget to put yourself first and love yourself.

CAPÍTULO VEINTE: F*CK TRUMP

Anderson and I had a great time in Israel. We both grew up Catholic, so it was cool to visit all the places that we learned about where Jesus roamed and went. We visited the Blue Mosque, the Wailing Wall, the old city, and the Stations of the Cross. We climbed the Masada at sunrise and visited the Dead Sea. We went into the West Bank to visit Ramallah, and Bethlehem, the Church of the Nativity where it is believed that Jesus was born, and the wall with all the art from Banksy that divides Israel from Palestine. We learned a lot and had a great hotel with breakfast included that had a view that overlooked Jerusalem.

Even though I often feel like I could travel full-time, there does come a point where you miss your home. You begin to miss your own bed, and you are ready to be back in your own culture, speaking your own language and living under rules and customs that are familiar. Two weeks was long enough to be in two foreign countries. We had seen a lot, and it is a trip that we will both never forget.

A week later, we arrived back in the United States and approached the USCIS customs line. As we moved through the line, a horrible image was glaring back at me. It was the face of the 45th President of the United States, Donald J. Trump. That orange hair and round red face was such a sore sight to look at. *What a horrible image to arrive home to,* I thought. He was the LAST person I wanted to see. Next to him on the wall was the commissioner of the USCIS and the American Flag.

Have you ever held a grudge against someone that you have never even met? Well, that was what I felt towards Donald Trump. I am not one to hold grudges, but it was Trump's fault that it took so long for Anderson to get his papers sorted out. It was all his fault that we had to wait a year and a half for him to be able to travel outside of the country. It was all his fault that we worried day in and day out, wondering if Anderson would be able to stay in the country legally. Donald Trump's distaste and negative attitude towards immigrants (even though his wife is one) kept us petrified for a year and a half, not knowing the outcome of what Anderson's legal status would be. Anderson had done everything legal since he arrived to the United States in 2014, including paying his taxes every year, but there was still a chance that he could have been denied his papers to stay in the country. We heard stories of so many other immigrants who were waiting legally, separated from family, children, and spouses that experienced even worse situations. And then there were those people stuck in jail with inhumane living conditions, separated from their families at the Mexico border.

Speaking of boundaries, Donald Trump has none. Still to this day, 5 years later, I cannot wrap my brain around why people voted for him and how he won. Oh, right, Russian interference. He has undone everything that President Obama worked so hard to rebuild and put in place after the recession of President Bush. I am not saying that Obama was perfect, but at least he was a decent human being that represented our country with dignity and respect. I truly believe that most of President Obama's decisions were made with good intentions. I also truly believe that every decision that Donald Trump has made is for the good of himself, and only himself (or his family), and the other rich people of the country.

Ever since Donald Trump announced that he was running for president, he has done and said anything that he wants, when he wants, and to whom he wants. Actually, I am pretty sure he has always been that way, but it is just more apparent now that he is the President of the United States and always in the spotlight.

It is sickening to see the leader of one of the greatest countries in the world use and abuse his power just to benefit himself and serve his wants and needs. It has been difficult to see a president overstep and cross every boundary there is, lie constantly, and disrespect and offend other world leaders, women, members of his cabinet and staff, with Ukraine, Iran, with immigrant families and their children, with Muslims, and the list goes on.

And most recently, on January 6, 2021, two weeks before his presidency term was over, he held a rally with his followers and encouraged them to storm the Capital. The Vice President, Mike Pence, and Congress were in session formally counting and registering the votes from the election that he lost, fair and square, that he convinced his followers was rigged. The disgrace and embarrassment of his actions made me so unproud to be American that day and throughout the last 4 years.

With the whole world watching, people died, and government member's lives were in danger. The president sat back and did nothing. He watched on TV, and even tweeted out a message to go after the Vice President, the man who supported him and all of his crazy actions throughout the last four years. Disgrace and disgust was all I could feel for that man.

Donald Trump tried to finagle his way into the election, and cause chaos afterwards, but thank God for our government's system of checks and balances so that the insanity and disrespect could not go on any longer.

Anderson and I went through the immigration line, grabbed our bags, and headed out into the Miami humidity. It was good to be home, but little did we know the year that was coming around the corner as we headed into 2020 and the coronavirus pandemic.

CAPÍTULO VEINTIUNO: CORONA WITH LIME

2020 changed the world forever. It will go down in the history books as one of, if not the WORST, year ever. As I am sitting here writing this, the current COVID-19 pandemic, also known as the coronavirus, is taking place all around me. I am quarantined in my home and only allowed to leave for groceries or to go to the doctor or the pharmacy. All non-essential businesses have been closed, and the world and its economy is at a standstill. Beaches and parks have been roped off and restaurants are only open for take-out, if they are open at all. No one knows what to do. The world is in a state of shock, and Miami Beach is a ghost town.

In December of 2019, shortly after we returned home from Spain and Israel, China reported their first case of COVID-19. It appears to have been carried from a bat that was at a wet market in China. Soon the virus was passed to thousands of Chinese people, which then turned into thousands of people in other countries due to travel and the contagiousness of this virus. Today, in August of 2021, there are more than 2.67 million cases tested positive for coronavirus and 4,264,820 deaths reported throughout 149 countries (Worldometer.com August 4, 2021). We just hit over 614,000 deaths in the United States alone.

Through all this madness, we have learned that this sickness spreads very easily, and today there are even various strains of the virus that are not being stopped even by the vaccines. One can be exposed and infected through the passing of germs from hanging out with other people, and the disease is sneaky in the sense that you can carry it without even feeling the symptoms and spread it to others. The danger of the virus affects mostly adults over age 65, people with illnesses and compromised immune systems, people with diabetes, cancer, and asthma or respiratory problems. Oh, wait, that is me.

I have had asthma since I was 8 years old. Every time I get sick, it goes to my chest. I randomly get wheezy, and if I do not use my inhaler, I can have an asthma attack. That has meant that I have needed to be extra careful and put boundaries up during this time like only leaving the house for necessities, only going to the grocery store one at a time, keeping my hands clean and distancing myself from groups. Really, just staying inside. I was quarantined for about a month inside without leaving my house, and many people around the world were really struggling with it, understandably.

Unfortunately, after over a year of being super safe, Anderson went to a barbecue with some friends that were visiting from Boston and became infected. Quickly it was passed to me, and even though I had received the first vaccine shot, I came down with the virus, too. Thankfully, it only lasted about a week and the symptoms were not serious enough to put either one of us in the hospital.

The world was completely shocked with the pandemic, and it started to take the virus more seriously at the beginning of March, 2020 when actor Tom Hanks and his wife both announced that they had tested positive for the coronavirus while on a trip to Australia. One by one, more "famous people" came forward to share that they had the virus. One of the bachelors from the television show tested positive. Andy Cohen, the head of the Bravo network, caught it. Various professional basketball players also tested positive, as well as the UK Prime

Minister, Boris Johnson, and the President of Harvard University and his wife. Donald Trump and his wife and son also got it. The sickness does not discriminate.

I have to admit, in the beginning, I did not take the coronavirus seriously. I was one of those people on the beach. I stayed a good distance away from crowds, but the beach was full of people because it was Spring Break in Miami. We went out to celebrate Anderson's birthday on March 16 and were around groups of people and went to restaurants that were full.

At the beginning of 2020, everyone was lost. People didn't know what to do. If you went outside, some people were dressed in full protection gear, gloves, and face masks. They looked like they were about to perform surgery at a hospital or ready for the apocalypse. Others were out on Spring Break and trying to take advantage of bars/restaurants that were still open. Others were laying on the parts of the beach that had some exposed sand that were not being guarded by the police even though the beaches were closed. Still, in 2021, the world is in shambles and trying to make sense out of all of this. Each person is handling it in their own way.

Due to the world being at a standstill, there have been many positive effects on the environment. For the first time in hundreds of years they have reported that you can see to the bottom of the waterways of Venice and dolphins have returned there. Air pollution has been heavily reduced because people have not been leaving their homes and driving. Factories are not running, and the majority of flights have been cancelled. The satellite photo from space is unrecognizable, because there isn't a thick cloud of pollution and you can actually see the Earth. I have heard people saying that this virus is Mother Earth's way of sending us all to our rooms for what we have done to the planet. Ain't that the truth?

LESSONS LEARNED

There are many lessons to be learned from the coronavirus. One is that the coronavirus does not discriminate, and yes, it can happen to you.

Two is that the world needs to slow down and value family and time with loved ones. People have had no choice but to stay at home and hang out together.

Three is that the media truly controls the world's state of being. I have tried my best to stay away from the news and negativity and just read what is needed on my phone. The media tries to purposely make people panic and live in a state of fear so that they stay glued to their TVs for more information.

Four, people are seeing how truly precious life is. While the majority of people affected by this disease are older, not just old people are dying. Children and middle-aged people have been affected too.

Five, people need to follow guidelines and limitations that are set in place in order to stop the virus from spreading. Boundaries in this situation are more important now than ever if we are going to truly stop spreading the virus and move forward so we can go back to normal, whatever that looks like moving forward.

Six, wash your hands, wear a mask, and love yourself.

Like I said at the beginning of this chapter, 2020 has changed the world forever. No one knows how long this will go on for, and the uncertainty of the future is difficult to think about. We have now been "home" for a year and a half, and we have not been able to travel to most countries until recently when the borders reopened.

As Tom Hanks and his wife requested of the world, please follow the rules of social distancing and take care of yourselves because the only Corona they want going forward, is a Corona with lime.

CONCLUSION

I hope you have enjoyed my stories and lessons that I have shared with you in this book. I want you to know that I set some boundaries while writing this book by making slight changes to some of the stories and characters. I also chose to leave out some serious stories that have happened in my life in order to set boundaries with those involved, and also to protect myself. Some stories are not meant to be told to the world, and I was able to still share the lessons and points that I wanted to get across in my examples through the stories that I did share without revealing some things that have occurred in my life.

I am leaving you with some information about boundary setting and a few questions for reflection. There is some space to journal or outline boundaries that you would like to improve on in your own life. Please reach out to discuss them or with any questions or thoughts that you want to share about setting boundaries. As difficult as it may seem, don't let fear stop you from setting limits. I promise you that the more you do it, the easier it becomes, and the better you will feel about yourself. Having the courage to do the right thing will build your character and strength. You are worth it.

I hope that you have walked away from this book with the following lessons:

*You are enough, just the way you are, so love yourself.

*I walked away from people, alcohol and situations to save myself.
*If I change, it is for myself because I want to be better.
*Live life to the fullest.
*Say no to people and things that don't serve you.
*Setting boundaries is a process and takes time.
*It is ok to say NO and not feel guilty about it.
*Setting boundaries will bring you happiness and freedom.
*Today I choose myself first.

Today I am free. Free from addiction. Free from a job I hate. Free from the entrapment of an abusive relationship. And I'm happy.

I had to stop drinking. I had to stop eating compulsively. I had to leave my job. And most importantly, I had to leave the toxic relationships. And today I'm happy.

The pain was real. The pain was deep. At times, I thought I couldn't go on. I was filled with shame and guilt, and wondered how I would be able to start over.

I've made it through to the other side. I learned to love again, and most importantly, I learned to love myself. I wouldn't change any of it, because today I am free.

Know that you are enough the way that you are and that your boundaries are valid. Listen to your gut, and don't be afraid to leave a job, a relationship, or any situation that no longer serves you. Life is too short to be unhappy, so love yourself.

Love,

Christine
Blondie With Borders

CAPÍTULO VEINTIDOS: BOUNDARIES AND HOW TO SET THEM

In order to live a happy life, setting physical and emotional boundaries is very important. Whether at work, with your relationships, your friends, or yourself, having boundaries in place leads to self-love and having good self-esteem. When you set a boundary, it causes a positive result or reaction from others which in turn makes you feel good about yourself. A direct result of setting limits is confidence and happiness with yourself and your relationships. Boundaries help build stability to avoid unhealthy relationships, burnout in your job/business, and are positive guidelines to teach others what is and is not acceptable when it comes to how you want to be treated.

In this book, I have shared various real-life situations and ways that I have had a lack of boundaries throughout my life. There are so many ways that I could have set boundaries with myself and others in all the situations that I shared. I have addressed issues, such as spending money, my relationship with food and alcohol, relationships with my exes, relationships with my family and friends, professional relationships, and boundary issues when traveling through years of therapy with an amazing counselor. I am so grateful to her for all the tough love and honesty that she has given me over the last 8 years.

I want to end the book by sharing some tips with you on how to set boundaries:

I. KNOW YOUR VALUES.

Ask yourself what is important to you, what goals you want to achieve, and what you desire to be the end result of the situation or relationship that you have. Keeping this at the forefront will help you remember why you want to set the boundary and also make it meaningful.

An example of this is, if I want to run a marathon, I must train for 3-4 months. Part of the training includes hydrating, running 5 times a week, and doing long runs on the weekends. This means limiting the amount of time that I go out with friends and going to bed early. Remembering that my end goal is to run the marathon, which is what is important to me, can help me at times when I want to go out with friends, or I don't feel like doing my runs or going to bed early. I remember my end goal, and it helps me stay on track.

2. COMMUNICATE YOUR BOUNDARIES CLEARLY

This is probably the most important step, because if you do not share the boundary with the other person or say no from the beginning, they will not know what your intention is, and they will likely violate it. If you lay the rules and guidelines down from the start, then there is a lower chance of it being violated.

An example of this is when I start working with a new client, I let them know from the beginning that my work schedule is 9 to

5, and that I do not work on Fridays or the weekend. (That's right—no Fridays either!). Sunday is the day that I spend with Anderson, and in December of 2020, I decided that I was going to give myself three-day weekends, because that is what I want.

If I let them know this from the beginning, they will not expect me to answer emails late at night or during the weekend. However, if I am not clear about this, then they will expect answers at all hours and times when I do not want to be working.

3. BRING UP A BOUNDARY VIOLATION RIGHT AWAY

After you have communicated a boundary that you have and someone does not respect it, it is important to call them out on it and bring it up immediately. They will likely continue violating the boundary if you do not say anything right away. Even if you have clearly stated your boundary from the beginning, people often forget it or do what they want anyway.

An example of this is when I worked at VIP Management and Michaela asked me if cigarettes bothered me. I told her yes, because I have asthma, and soon I was going home smelling like cigarette smoke and with breathing problems, because I allowed her to continue to smoke in front of me without telling her again that it bothered me.

4. CREATE STRUCTURE AT WORK OR WITH SPENDING

If you have a boss or coworker who tends to go off-topic and make meetings longer than needed, show up with an agenda, and let them know the items you want to cover in the 30 minutes that you have.

Take the focus off of you and try not to say, "I am stressed and don't have time."

It is helpful if you show them how it benefits them, so if you say, "If I spend a long time at this meeting, then I will not have enough time to work on project X."

Similarly, it is helpful if you set up a structure with your money, like a budget, or look at your finance statements frequently to know what money is coming in and where your money is being spent. Having structure or a system with money in place will allow you to stay out of debt.

5. BE PREPARED FOR PEOPLE TO NOT RESPECT YOUR BOUNDARIES

You can set boundaries, and people will still do what they want. They will test you and try to cross them. It is helpful to imagine your boundaries being crossed and also having a plan in place of how you will handle the situation when that happens. If you do that ahead of time, you will be prepared to respond in the way that you want and not based on your emotions at that time.

For example, if your boss contacts you on Sunday asking you to work on a project, you can imagine this happening ahead of time and already have thought through what your response will be. You can have an automatic message go up on your emails on the weekend saying that you will respond to any emails on Monday. That way whoever emails you on the weekend knows when to expect a response.

6. JUST SAY, "NO."

I think we often forget that "No" is a full sentence. There is no need for any explanation, and no reason to feel guilty, no is just no. I think women especially have a hard time with saying no in certain situations. As natural caretakers and caring people, sometimes we can get caught up in our emotions and feel guilty for putting ourselves before others.

However, the real truth is, if we do not put ourselves first, we will not be available to take care of others. If I do not wake up and do my morning meditation, I likely will not be in the same mood or mindset for the rest of the day to take care of myself and my husband. If I do not get my workout in, I can become overweight and emotionally unhappy, which in turn will have an effect on my family and those I work with. Everything has a ripple effect.

I am also setting an example for those around me. Children learn behaviors from their parents and are always watching. If I create a routine for myself to wake up, meditate, and workout, my child will know that as being "normal," and they will have a better chance of also having a healthier lifestyle.

Finally, if your boundaries are being violated in any way, I encourage you to stop and take a look at how you can push the reset button. Boundaries take time and practice to set in place, and most of your boundaries will be tested at some time. The process of learning how to create and set boundaries does not happen overnight, however it does get easier the more you set and enforce them.

Try to use your experiences as a way to learn and see where you can improve your boundary setting. If you are in any toxic environment, whether it be a relationship, a work setting, or deep into debt, I encourage you to face it head on and see what you can do to change it. Leaving any toxic environment is setting a boundary in itself by saying "no more" and simply removing yourself. Putting yourself first is setting boundaries to the world and, of course, loving yourself.

BOUNDARY QUESTIONS FOR REFLECTION:

1. What are the boundaries that I already have set in place in my life in the areas of work, love relationships, family, money, job, and at home?

2. Write down 5 boundaries that I want to change or set moving forward?

3. Why do I want to set these boundaries? What are my goals? Why are they important to me?

4. How will I create structure to make sure I follow through on my new boundaries?

5. How am I going to communicate these boundaries to those involved? Write a plan.

6. What will I do when these boundaries are violated? How will I react and what will I do to reinforce my boundary?

REFLECTIONS

ACKNOWLEDGEMENTS

First, I would like to thank everyone who has loved and supported me along my journey to learning who Christine is through the process of becoming Blondie With Borders, so that I can live a healthier, happier life.

I would like to thank Candis and Sol, my two weekly writing partners. We spent endless weekday mornings sitting and writing our books while keeping each other accountable. When the coronavirus hit, we stayed committed and wrote many mornings in silence on Zoom. Just knowing that you were there writing your own books helped encourage me and carry me along. Thank you for sharing your lessons learned, your thoughts, and your reflections each week as we supported each other on this journey.

Thank you to Vivian Olodun, who helped me believe that I could write this book. Thank you for hosting your free book-writing sessions to teach others the behind the scenes of self-publishing, and for listening to my ideas and sharing your own in order to make this book come to fruition.

Thank you to Shawn Brooks, who encouraged me to write my book and reminded me when I was afraid that I am worthy of sharing my story with the world so that I can help others through the lessons I have learned.

Thank you to my cousin, Aimee, who went through many experiences with me, both personally and through travel, and for encouraging me to share my crazy stories by planting the idea of 'writing a book someday.'

Thank you to Wanderson for always being by my side. Thank you to my family and loved ones who went through and supported my growing pains over the years. Thank you for your unending love, patience, and guidance to help me become the strong woman I am today, Blondie With Borders.